ISBN 978-1-334-56454-3
PIBN 10730040

YELLOW FEVER COMMISSION

(WEST AFRICA).

FOURTH AND FINAL REPORT.

Price 5/- nett.

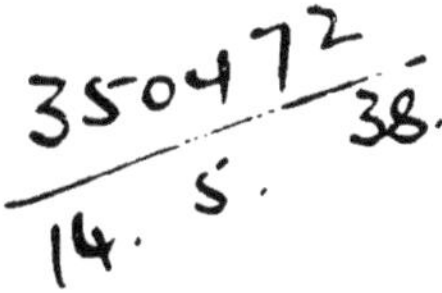

PUBLISHED BY:

J. & A. CHURCHILL, 7, GREAT MARLBOROUGH STREET, LONDON, W.

1916

TABLE OF CONTENTS.

FOURTH AND FINAL REPORT

OF

THE YELLOW FEVER COMMISSION (WEST AFRICA.)

PART I.

WORK OF THE COMMISSION.

The period of three years for which the Commission were appointed having expired, it becomes their duty to present a Fourth and Final Report of their proceedings.

2. Since August, 1914, the work upon which they have been engaged has been seriously hindered by the outbreak of war.

The atmosphere which war creates renders research, unless in subjects directly connected therewith, almost impossible. This is in part due to the fact that nearly all who are qualified for research desire to undertake work of a more active kind on behalf of their country.

In the West African Dependencies it became necessary to recall the members of the West African Medical Staff who were acting as appointed Investigators of the Commission to other duties, and it was not found possible to replace them.

3. Owing to these circumstances the Commission are compelled, with regret, to bring the enquiry upon which they were engaged to an end, whilst many of the problems under investigation are still unsolved.

This is the more unfortunate as, after one of those periods of quiescence, which are so characteristic of the course of this disease, a fresh outbreak occurred in September and October, 1915, at Onitsha, Nigeria, where there were two cases in natives, one of which was fatal; at Burutu, a fatal case in a native; and at a camp known as "Engenni Concessions," on Engenni River, twenty miles from Degema, where seven cases occurred in natives, of which two were fatal. From Kaduna, one fatal case in a European is also reported.

Possibly, at some later period, when the conditions are more favourable, these researches may be resumed and carried to a successful conclusion.

4. The continuity of attendance at the meetings of the Commission has been from time to time interrupted by the calls made upon its members for service under the Government abroad. Thus Professor Simpson was absent on an important mission to East Africa from May, 1913, to January, 1914. The services of Sir William Leishman have not been available since the outbreak of war. Sir Ronald Ross was engaged on a mission to Cyprus in March and April, 1913, and on military duty in Egypt from July to the end of November, 1915. Dr. Andrew Balfour, who was added to the Commission in November, 1914, was called upon for service in the Eastern Mediterranean in July, 1915.

5. The Commission were appointed by Mr. Secretary Harcourt in January, 1913, with the following reference:—

"To study the nature and the relative frequency of the fevers occurring among Europeans, natives and others in West Africa, especially with regard to Yellow Fever and other non-malarial fevers in that country."

6. The Commission have held seventy-four meetings, including several laboratory meetings, and have also personally carried out laboratory examinations in connection with material sent home by Investigators and others. They have had interviews with the following gentlemen, who kindly attended to place their knowledge at the disposal of the Commission:—

J. B. Tombleson, M.B., B.Ch. (Oxon), late W.A.M.S.

David Thompson, M.B., Ch.B. (Edin.), D.P.H. (Cantab.).

T. E. Rice, L.S.A. (Lond.), D.P.H. (Ireland), W.A.M.S.; Principal Medical Officer, Gold Coast.

H. S. Coghill, M.B., Ch.B. (Edin.), W.A.M.S.; Assistant Bacteriologist, Medical Research Institute, Lagos.

H. M. Hänschell, M.R.C.S. (Eng.), L.R.C.P. (Lond.), late W.A.M.S.

Lieut.-Col. A. Lisle Webb, C.M.G., R.A.M.C.

E. A. Chartres, F.R.C.S. (Ireland), D.P.H. (Ireland), W.A.M.S.; Deputy Principal Medical Officer, Nigeria (Northern Provinces).

Harald Seidelin, M.D. (Copenhagen).

Major W. H. G. H. Best, L.R.C.S., L.R.C.P. (Ireland), W.A.M.S., R.A.M.C. (S.R.); Principal Medical Officer, Nigeria (Southern Provinces).

G. E. H. Le Fanu, M.B., Ch.B. (Aberd.), W.A.M.S.; Medical Officer, Gold Coast.

A. Connal, M.D., Ch.B. (Glas.), D.P.H. (Cantab.), W.A.M.S.; Director of the Medical Research Institute, Lagos.

J. M. O'Brien, M.R.C.S. (Eng.), L.R.C.P. (Lond.), W.A.M.S.; Medical Officer, Gold Coast.

Surgeon-General Sir Charles Purdey Lukis, M.B. (Lond.), F.R.C.S. (Eng.), K.C.S.I., K.H.P.; Director-General, I.M.S.

A. E. Horn, M.D., B.Sc. (Lond.), W.A.M.S.; Senior Medical Officer, Gambia.

G. G. Butler, M.B., B.C. (Cantab.), M.R.C.S. (Eng.), L.R.C.P. (Lond.), W.A.M.S.; Medical Officer, Sierra Leone.

Lieutenant-Colonel J. C. B. Statham, C.M.G., R.A.M.C.

J. E. L. Johnston, M.B., B.S. (Lond.), M.R.C.S. (Eng.), L.R.C.P. (Lond.), W.A.M.S.; Medical Officer, Nigeria.

S. T. Darling, M.D.; Chief of the Laboratory, Ancon Hospital, Panama Canal Zone.

Surgeon-General W. C. Gorgas, Medical Corps, United States Army; Chief Sanitary Officer, Isthmian Canal Commission.

R. Mugliston, M.R.C.S. (Eng.), L.R.C.P. (Lond.), W.A.M.S.; Medical Officer, Gold Coast.

F. Beringer, M.R.C.S. (Eng.), L.R.C.P. (Lond.), D.P.H. (Ireland), W.A.M.S.; Sanitary Officer, Sierra Leone.

F. G. Hopkins, M.D., B.Ch. (Dublin), W.A.M.S.; late Principal Medical Officer, Gold Coast.

T. Hood, M.R.C.S. (Eng.), L.R.C.P. (Lond.), W.A.M.S.; Director of the Medical and Sanitary Service of Nigeria.

J. C. M. Bailey, M.D. (Lond.), M.R.C.S. (Eng.), L.R.C.P. (Lond.), W.A.M.S.; Medical Officer, Nigeria.

S C. O. Pontifex, Collector of Customs, Nigeria.

D. Mackinnon, M.B., Ch.B., D.P.H. (Edin.), W.A.M.S.; Medical Officer, Nigeria.

A. Hutton, M.B., Ch.B. (Aberd.), W.A.M.S.; Medical Officer, Nigeria.

J. W. Collett, L.R.C.S., L.R.C.P. (Edin.), L.F.P.S. (Glas.), W.A.M.S.; Provincial Medical Officer, Nigeria.

E. W. GRAHAM, M.B., C.M. (Glas.), W.A.M.S.; Provincial Medical Officer, Gold Coast.

J. A. PICKELS, M.B., B.S. (Lond.), D.P.H. (Liverpool), W.A.M.S.; Senior Sanitary Officer, Nigeria (Southern Provinces).

J. W. SCOTT MACFIE, M.B., Ch.B. (Edin.), W.A.M.S.; Pathologist, Gold Coast.

T. M. R. LEONARD, L.R.C.S., L.R.C.P. (Edin.), L.F.P.S. (Glas.), W.A.M.S.; Medical Officer, Nigeria.

A. W. BACOT, F.E.S., Entomologist to the Lister Institute of Preventive Medicine.

W. E. DEEKS, M.D.; Chief of the Medical Clinic, Ancon Hospital.

Major PERRY, Medical Corps, United States Army; Sanitary Department, Panama Canal Zone.

W. H. A. GORDON HALL, M.B., C.M. (Edin.), W.A.M.S.; Provincial Medical Officer, Nigeria.

Dr. FELIX PAEZ, Director of the Medical Department of the Hospital Ruiz, Ciudad Bolivar, Venezuela.

7. The various steps taken by the Commission to organise their work are fully stated in the First Report and need not be repeated. They included the appointment of Investigators detailed for work at various places on the West Coast of Africa. A list of the Investigators is given below, showing where they worked and the reports which they have furnished, with references to such of them as have been published, either in the Volumes of Reports issued by the Commission or elsewhere: —

Name, Title and Place of Work.	Reference to Report.
Lieutenant-Colonel J. C. B. STATHAM, C.M.G., M.R.C.S., (Eng.), L.R.C.P. (London), D.P.H. (R.C.P.S., Eng. and London); R.A.M.C.; at Freetown, Sierra Leone.*	I.R. Vol. II., pp. 353 to 387.
G. G. BUTLER, M.A., M.B., B.C., (Cantab.), M.R.C.S., (Eng.), L.R.C.P., (London); W.A.M.S.; at Freetown	I.R. Vol. II., pp. 389 to 417.
J. M. DALZIEL, M.D., C.M. (Edin.), B.Sc., Public Health (Edin.), D.T.M. (Liverpool); W.A.M.S.; at Freetown.	I.R. Vol. II., pp. 527 to 579.
W. B. JOHNSON, M.B., B.Sc. (London), F.R.C.S. (Eng.), L.R.C.P. (London); W.A.M.S.; at Freetown.	Do. do.
A. W. BACOT, F.E.S., Entomologist to the Lister Institute of Preventive Medicine; at Freetown.	Investigators' Reports, Vol. III.†

*Lieut.-Col. (then Major) Statham resigned his position as Investigator shortly after his appointment, but continued to do similar work and to collaborate with Dr. Butler in a private capacity.

†Not yet published.

Name, Title and Place of Work—*continued.*	Reference to Report—*continued.*
H. S. Coghill, M.B., Ch.B., (Edin.), D.T.M. & H. (Cantab.); W.A.M.S.; at Sekondi and Accra, and in the Northern Territories, Gold Coast.	I.R. Vol. II., pp. 653 to 730.
H. M. Hänschell, M.R.C.S. (Eng.), L.R.C.P. (London), D.T.M. (Liverpool); late Senior Demonstrator, London School of Tropical Medicine; late W.A.M.S.; at Sekondi, Gold Coast.	Do. do.
G. E. H. Le Fanu, M.B., C.M. (Aberdeen), D.T.M. (Liverpool); W.A.M.S.; at Accra and Quittah, Gold Coast.	I.R. Vol. II., pp. 581 to 594; I.R. Vol. III.*
Harald Seidelin, M.D. (Copenhagen); (late) Director, Yellow Fever Bureau, Liverpool; at Accra, Gold Coast, and Lagos, Nigeria.	I.R. Vol. II., pp. 421 to 478; 483 to 526.
A. Hutton, M.B., Ch.B. (Aberdeen), D.T.M. & H. (Cantab.); (late) W.A.M.S.; at Accra, Gold Coast.	—
†T. M. R. Leonard, L.R.C.S., L.R.C.P. (Edin.), L.F.P.S. (Glas.): W.A.M.S.; at Lagos, Nigeria.	I.R. Vol. I., pp. 207 to 316.
†J. W. Scott-Magpie, B.A. (Cantab.), M.B., Ch.B. (Edin.); D.T.M. (Liverpool); W.A.M.S.; Pathologist, Accra; at the Medical Research Institute, Lagos, Nigeria.	Proceedings of the Royal Soeiety ot Medicine, Vol. III., 1914, (Medical Section), pp. 49-67 (also published in the Yellow Fever Bulletin, Vol. III. No. 2, pp. 121-144).
J. E. L. Johnston, M.B., B.S. (Lond.), M.R.C.S. (Eng.), L.R.C.P. (Lond.), D.T.M. & H. (Cantab.); W.A.M.S.; at the Medical Research Institute, Lagos, Nigeria.	Do. do. and I.R. Vol. II., pp. 595 to 652.
†(Temporary) Captain E. J. Wyler, M.D., B.S. (Lond.), M.R.C.S. (Eng.), L.R.C.P. (Lond.); R.A.M.C. (late W.A.M.S.); at Lagos, Abeokuta, Warri. Forcados and Lagos, Nigeria.	I.R. Vol. I. pp. 2 to 206.
†A. Connal, M.D., Ch.B. (Glas.), D.P.H., D.T.M. & H. (Cantab.); W.A.M.S.; Director of the Medical Research Institute, Lagos, Nigeria; at the Institute.	I.R. Vol. II., pp. 421 to 478: 595 to 652.

*Not yet published.

†These gentlemen were not definitely appointed Investigators under the Commission, but carried out work on the same lines. Dr. Connal was the appointed officer through whose hands "case cards" and other records passed from Nigeria to the Commission, and blood films and pathological material from suspected cases were examined at the Medical Research Institute under his supervision.

8. The Commission are also indebted to the following members of the Medical Profession who have assisted in their work in various ways, either in West Africa or at home:—

Sir PATRICK MANSON, G.C.M.G., M.D. (Aberd.), F.R.C.P. (Lond.), F.R.S.

Lieutenant-Colonel S. L. CUMMINS, C.M.G., M.D. (R.U.I.), R.A.M.C.

Lieutenant-Colonel D. HARVEY, M.D. (Glas.), R.A.M.C.

(Temporary) Lieutenant-Colonel C. M. WENYON, M.B. B.S., B.Sc. (Lond.), R.A.M.C.; Wellcome Bureau of Scientific Research.

H. M. TURNBULL, M.D., B.Ch. (Oxon.), M.R.C.S. (Eng.), L.R.C.P. (Lond.); Director of the Pathological Institute, London Hospital.

J. W. CROPPER, M.B., Ch.B., M.Sc. (Liverpool), M.R.C.S. (Eng.), L.R.C.P. (Lond.), Lister Institute of Preventive Medicine.

(Temporary) Captain A. LUNDIE, M.B., Ch.B. (Edin.), B.Sc. (St. Andrews), R.A.M.C. (late W.A.M.S.).

(Temporary) Lieutenant J. C. THOMSON, M.B., Ch.B. (Edin.), R.A.M.C.; Lecturer in Protozoology, London School of Tropical Medicine.

A. C. STEVENSON, M.B. (Lond.), M.R.C.S. (Eng.), L.R.C.P. (Lond.); Wellcome Bureau of Scientific Research.

E. F. WARD, M.D., B.Ch., B.A.O. (Belfast); W.A.M.S.

M. E. MACGREGOR, B.A. (Cantab.); Wellcome Bureau of Scientific Research.

9. The Commission have already presented three Reports, and have published two volumes* containing Reports received from appointed Investigators and others. (A third volume is in the press.)

These volumes contain many papers of great interest, and it is believed that they form a valuable addition to our knowledge of Yellow Fever, and in a lesser degree also of Malaria and other diseases.

10. The First Report was presented in order to make clear the scope of the reference and the steps which had already been taken to give effect to the instructions.

This step appeared to be desirable, in order that there might not be overlapping, should it be decided to appoint another Commission

* The full reference is as follows: "Yellow Fever Bureau Bulletin, Yellow Fever Commission (West Africa). Reports on questions connected with the Investigation of Non-Malarial Fevers in West Africa." These volumes are here referred to thus: "I.R., vol.——."

to consider the possibility that, on the opening of the Panama Canal, Yellow Fever might be carried to countries in which hitherto it had been unknown.

11. In their Second Report the Commission dealt chiefly with the history of Yellow Fever in relation to the West African Colonies. The evidence adduced to prove that the disease had been present in one or other Colony upon the Coast for at least 130 years has been accepted as justifying that conclusion.

It was shown that during this period its activity had been subject to great variations, and that in every Colony, during recurring periods, often of prolonged duration, there was no record of the occurrence of an epidemic amongst the European inhabitants, although during the years comprised within these intervals cases of a suspicious character had often occurred, which had been recorded under one or other of the numerous euphemisms commonly employed in the past to hide the presence of Yellow Fever.

In some Colonies these intervals had in later times become fewer and briefer, as the records became more complete, and the necessity for constant attention to sanitary measures more appreciated by the Government concerned.

12. The Third Report of the Commission was almost entirely devoted to the various questions connected with the claim of Dr. Harald Seidelin to have discovered the virus of Yellow Fever, in the form of bodies to which he had given the name of *Paraplasma flavigenum*.

As the result of researches undertaken or suggested by the Commission, evidence was obtained which led them to conclude that the bodies in question had no pathological significance, and that they were in no way specially connected with Yellow Fever.

The Commission are of opinion that the facts therein set out are conclusive against Dr. Seidelin's claim.

13. This Fourth and Final Report is divided into five parts, of which the foregoing sections constitute Part I.

Part II. deals with the presence of various fevers among natives and Europeans, in West Africa, excluding Yellow Fever.

Part III. is devoted especially to Yellow Fever.

Part IV. contains suggestions for further research and in regard to quarantine, the general conclusions at which the Commission have arrived, and also references to the services of Investigators and others.

Part V.—Appendices.

At the head of Parts II., III. and IV. a synopsis is given of the contents of those parts of the Report.

PART II.

THE PRESENCE OF VARIOUS FEVERS AMONG NATIVES AND EUROPEANS, EXCLUDING YELLOW FEVER.

SYNOPSIS.

One of the problems to which the attention of the Investigators appointed by the Commission was specially directed was stated thus:—

"Do the following diseases occur in West Africa?
"If so, to what extent?
"(*a*) Dengue Fever.
"(*b*) Pappataci Fever.
"(*c*) Typhus.
"(*d*) Rocky Mountain Fever.
"(*e*) Double continued Fever.
"(*f*) Typhoid.
"(*g*) Paratyphoid.
"(*h*) Undulant Fever (formerly Malta Fever).
"(*i*) Para-undulant Fever.
"(*j*) Cerebro-spinal Fever."

Another problem was:—

"The nature of the fevers which have been termed—
"(*a*) Bilious Remittent Fever.
"(*b*) Malignant Bilious Remittent Fever.
"(*c*) Inflammatory, Endemial or Acclimatising Fever.
"(*d*) Hyperpyrexial Fever.
"(*e*) Three Days' Fever.
"(*f*) Seven Days' Fever.
"(*g*) Low Fever.
"(*h*) Febricula."

The Commission cannot claim to have made, through their Investigators, an exhaustive study of these various types of fever; that part of the work has been rendered incomplete by the events to which reference has already been made.

A considerable amount of evidence as regards the occurrence in West Africa of some of these fevers has however been obtained and will now be stated.

SECTION I.

DENGUE, PAPPATACI FEVER, THREE DAYS' FEVER AND SEVEN DAYS' FEVER.

Dengue.

There has certainly been no epidemic of Dengue Fever on the West Coast during the period covered by the work of the Commission, and in the absence of such a clear indication of the presence of that disease it is advisable to speak with some reserve as to the nature of the cases which have presented signs suggesting such a diagnosis.

Vol. II., 353—386. The second volume of the Investigators' Reports contains an account by Lieutenant-Colonel J. C. B. Statham, C.M.G., R.A.M.C., of a series of 800 medical pyrexias investigated by him at Sierra Leone in 1912 and 1913. In all 1,100 cases were investigated.

Colonel Statham, in discussing the possible nature of 70 cases of undiagnosed fever where no malaria parasites were found in the blood, writes as follows (p. 381):—

> "*Pappataci, Dengue, Three-day Fever and Seven-day Fever.*— * * * * * * The majority of the remaining cases were, I think, from clinical and bacteriological grounds, cases of malaria where the parasites had been missed, either owing to a single blood examination only having been made, or to the great scarcity of parasites, a condition which one so often notices in subtertian malarial infection out here. There remain other cases where the most complete search on successive days failed to reveal malaria parasites, and some of these cases may have belonged to the group of diseases mentioned above.
>
> "The sporadic rather than epidemic nature of the cases, and the absence of rashes, conjunctival injection, and joint affections, appears to negative pappataci fever, or dengue in the epidemic form, but some of the cases may have been of the nature of sporadic dengue or seven-days' fever, if these are clinical entities. * * * * * * Though *Simuliidæ* and *Chironomidæ* abound in Sierra Leone, I have never met with nor heard of the *Phlebotomus pappatasii.*"

One case in Colonel Statham's series is classed as "? Dengue or exanthem." The patient was a European woman, age 35, resident in Freetown, who was taken ill on August 29th, 1913, and when seen on the following day had a temperature of 102°F. She complained of fulness in the head, pains and aches all over the body, slight sore throat, dyspepsia and buzzing in the ears. The tongue was furred, but with a slight strawberry appearance. The face was flushed, there was no conjunctival injection, no jaundice, vomiting or diarrhœa. A slight cloud of albumen was present in the urine. The pulse varied between 86 and 94. The temperature fell to 100°F. on the third day and remained almost steady at that level for five days; on the seventh day it became normal. An erythematous rash was present on the face, chest, back and arms; it did not resemble any specific rash. Four days later, 4/10/13, a punctate rash appeared over the whole of the body, and was especially marked on the forearms, palms and fingers. This rash faded on the following day, and was almost immediately followed by a third rash of a diffuse morbiliform character. This also lasted one day, and after it the skin peeled. The patient stated that she always had a rash after a chill. Two blood examinations for malaria parasites were negative.

I.R. Vol. p. 371 (No. 71.)

In the house in which the patient lived many *Culex* and *Stegomyia* were found and three other cases of fever had occurred amongst the inmates.

The evidence afforded by a single case of this kind is obviously insufficient to establish the fact that Dengue fever is to be met with in Sierra Leone.

Dr. Hutton, one of the Investigators of the Commission, stated in an interview:—

> "One case of dengue had been diagnosed in the Gold Coast just before he went there.
>
> "The patient was a Mrs. H. (she left hospital a few days after Dr. Hutton's arrival), who had been a nurse, and recognised that the rash was quite different from that of scarlet fever, etc. Dr. O'Brien and Dr. Connal had diagnosed the ease, and their diagnosis had been confirmed by Dr. Dowse, who had experience of dengue in Fiji."

A case which was classified by the Commission as "Possibly Dengue" occurred at Naraguta, in Northern Nigeria, in April, 1913.

The clinical record is, briefly, as follows:—

26.* "Mr. A., Surveyor, ? age, had been feeling unwell for a day or two, with aches in his bones. When seen on April 23rd he complained of headache and a rash. The eyes were deeply injected. Face flushed, tongue coated; temperature, 102° F. The whole body was covered with a profuse scarlatiniform rash, slightly marked on forehead, absent on palms and soles. The rash was slightly rough to the touch, and the affected skin was tender.

"April 24th. Temperature, 103° F.

"April 25th. Temperature, 99° F. Rash partially faded. Eyes still injected.

"April 28th. Rash disappeared. Temperature normal. No desquamation."

A second case of a similar nature, also classified as "Possibly Dengue," occurred at Naraguta, in November, 1913.

27. The following are the notes of this case:—

"Mr. B., Mine Manager.

"On Nov. 16th complained of severe pains in body and legs, especially on movement. Could with difficulty get out of bed.

"Temperature 102° F. at 7 p.m.

"For the next two days pains grew less, but temperature was still raised in the evening.

"Nov. 19th. Scarlatiniform rash appeared first on chest, abdomen, and back. Eyes injected. Face flushed. Temperature, 99° F. at 6 p.m.

"Nov. 20th. Rash had extended to arms and legs, and was very profuse on body, slightly marked on forehead. Eyes deeply injected. Palms and soles free, but he complained of head and tenderness in them. Rash generally was tender to touch and heat. There was some tenderness of glands in axilla and groin. Temperature, 99° F.

"Liver and spleen normal.

"Urine contained no albumen.

"Nov. 22nd. Rash much faded. Temperature normal.

"Nov. 23rd. Rash entirely disappeared. No signs of desquamation.

"Blood showed no parasites.

"Mononuclear ... ... 21 per cent.

"Eosinophiles ... ... 5 " " "

---

* The numbers quoted in the margin, where no other reference is given, are those assigned to the cases by the Investigators (at Lagos and elsewhere), through whose hands the records passed to the Commission. For an account of the system adopted see the First Report of the Commission (page 33, etc.).

Pappataci Fever.

In a synopsis of cases of fever reported from Nigeria to the L. 17.
Medical Research Institute, Yaba, S. Nigeria, up to July 22nd, 1913, L. 18. L. 19.
Dr. J. W. Scott Macfie, the Acting Director, summarizes four cases of Pappataci fever, all of which occurred in Europeans, thus:—

"*Pappataci Fever.*

"Three cases of fever reported from Ibadan (Nos. 17, 18 and 19), and one (No. 20) from Lagos, are suggestive of pappataci fever. These cases were characterised by the sudden onset and the short duration of the fever; pains in the back and limbs; headache; nausea or vomiting, and digestive disorders; and pharyngitis. The pulse was slow, but of good quality. There was neither tenderness nor enlargement of the liver and spleen. Albuminuria was not present; and the blood was negative in the cases in which examinations were made. In two cases convalescence was prolonged, in the other two it was brief. In this respect the latter cases (Nos. 18 and 19) differed from typical pappataci fever. A history of bites from sand-flies accompanied the cases. It can scarcely be doubted, therefore, that these were cases of pappataci fever.

Table of symptoms in four cases, probably Pappataci Fever.

Case No.	17	18	19	20
Onset, sudden...	+	+	+	+
Fever, 1 to 2 days	+	+	...	+
Convalescence, slow	+	−	...	+
Headache	+	+	+	+
Severe pains in the back, loins, &c.	+	+	+	+
Eyes injected	...	...	+	+
Vomiting and digestive disorders	+	+	...	+
Pharyngitis and tonsilitis ...	...	+	+	+
Tongue, tip red	+	+	...	+
Slow pulse of good quality ...	+	+	+	+
Slow pulse in convalescence ...	+	+	...	+
Albuminuria	−	−	−	−
Blood—Malarial parasites ...	−	...	−	−

+ : present; − : absent; ... : no observation.

"A case (No. 21) reported from Ebute-Metta, near Lagos, should also, perhaps, be included here. With regard to the occurrence of sand-flies, *Culicoides grahami* is the only species known to occur at Lagos; but I believe that the Entomologist to the Agricultural Department has recently taken specimens belonging to both the genera *Phlebotomus* and *Simulium* at Ibadan."

One of these cases was reported by Dr. T. W. Russell Leonard, as follows: —

"CASE OF PAPPATACI FEVER.

"*No.* 20. *Name.*—D. L. D.

"*Sex.*—Male.

"*Age.*—23 years.

"*Nationality.*—British.

"*Occupation.*—Assistant Auditor.

"*Date of admission.*—21st May, 1913.

"*Date of discharge.*—26th May, 1913.

"*Diagnosis.*—Pappataci fever (sand-fly fever, three days' fever).

"*History.*—Patient states that he was apparently quite well and fit up to 10 p.m. on the night of the 20th of May. At 10.30, after going to bed, he began to have a severe frontal headache, accompanied by aches and pains in the muscles of the legs, thighs and loins. Later he experienced pains in the epigastrium, which were followed by vomiting, accompanied by several profuse watery motions; his bowels had previously been constipated. His temperature rose, but he had no thermometer to register it. He spent a very restless night, the vomiting and diarrhœa continued on and off, the headache got worse, and the muscular pains increased; so at 5 a.m. he sent for a doctor, and Dr. Wyler went and saw him and sent him into hospital at 7.30 a.m., the 21st.

"*Condition on admission.*—Patient complains of severe headache, sore throat, muscular pains in the leg, thigh and lumbar muscles; the vomiting had stopped.

"Face was flushed, the conjunctivæ of both eyes were red and injected, the injection appearing as a red band passing across the eye and corresponding to palpebral fissure.

"*Alimentary system.*—Tongue is coated, with clean tip. Pharynx is congested. Tonsils also congested and red. Complains of soreness when swallowing. Stomach is irritable. Epigastrium is tender on pressure. Liver is normal. Spleen also normal, no tenderness on palpation. Vomiting had been very troublesome, but had now stopped. Had several watery motions through the night accompanied by pains in the epigastrium. The motions were yellow and watery, otherwise normal.

"*Circulatory system*—Area of cardiac dulness is normal. Heart sounds are normal in character. Pulse rate 78 mt.

"*Nervous system.*—Headache pronounced, felt in the frontal region.

"Pains in the muscles of the leg, thigh, of both lower extremities, and also in the lumbar muscles. The pains were increased on pressure. There was pronounced tenderness of both peroneal nerves.

"*Urinary system.*—Urine was passed freely; on examination high coloured. Acid reaction. Sp. gr. 1,030. No albumen.

"*Blood examination.*—No malaria fever parasites found. Red cells normal in appearance.

"Leucocyte count: polymorph., 80 per cent.; l. mononuclear, 10 per cent.; lymphocyte, 10 per cent.; eosinophiles, nil.

"*Other systems.*—The skin over both lower extremities shows the marks of numerous bites by sand-flies, the patient stating that he was bitten chiefly at night.

"The patient is a new arrival in West Africa, and has never been in the tropics before; he takes quinine regularly and uses a mosquito-net at night.

"*21st May.*—The pulse rate on admission was 78 mt., but during the day there was pronounced bradycardia. the pulse rate at 12 noon being 56 mt., and faintly dicrotic; temperature being 98°. At 6 p.m. the pulse was 52, and at 8 p.m. it was 64 mt. The muscular pains continued, but the frontal decreased in severity under the treatment.

"*22nd May.*—Patient had a good night, slept well, and feels more comfortable this morning. Temperature is 97·2°, pulse 50 mt., still faintly dicrotic. At 11 a.m. the pulse was 48 mt., and at 6 p.m. it was 50 mt. The muscular pains are much easier, but the peroneal nerves are still very sensitive to pressure. Appetite is poor; bowels moved once. The pharynx is still sore on swallowing, and is red and congested in appearance.

"*23rd May.*—Patient passed a good night, feels much better this morning. Temperature is 97·4°, pulse 62 mt. At 10 a.m. pulse rate was 48 mt., and at 8 p.m. was 64. Muscular pains are very much lessened, but still present on pressure; the peronii nerves are also still sensitive to pressure.

"*24th May.*—Temperature 97°, in the evening it was 98°. Patient had a good night and feels very much improved. The muscles are not painful, but are on firm pressure. Pulse rate still shows a pronounced bradycardia—at 9 a.m. 58, at 12 noon 56, at 4 p.m. 64, and at 8 p.m. it was 70 mt.

"*25th May.*—Patient slept well, and feels quite well this morning. No pains in the muscles or nerves. Pulse rate at 9 a.m. 62, at 12 noon 58, and at 6 p.m. it was 60 mt.

"*26th May.*—Patient feels quite well, appetite improved, bowels regular. Pulse rate was 75 mt. at 9 a.m., and in the afternoon it was 75 mt. Discharged from hospital."

Name, D. L. D., British. *Sex*, Male. *Age*, 23 years.
Occupation, Assistant Auditor. *Disease*, Pappataci Fever.

In Appendix A of Dr. T. M. Russell Leonard's "Report on certain outbreaks of Yellow Fever in Lagos, 1913, and January and February, 1914," the following reference to Pappataci fever occurs:— I.R. Vol. I. pp. 207—3c (p. 299).

"In pappataci fever, of which I have had several cases here in Lagos, we also have a pyrexia ushered in with violent headache, chiefly frontal and orbital, aching pains in the muscles of the limbs, epigastralgia, pain in the peroneal and intercostal nerves, flushed face with conjunctival injection, the injection taking the form of a red band across the eyes. Vomiting and diarrhœa are present in most cases and are often the initial symptoms. An important symptom is the presence of a pharyngitis; epistaxis very often occurs. The temperature and pulse both rise and, as the temperature falls, a typical bradycardia is established, with a slow return to normal conditions during convalescence. The urine is high coloured, but contains no albumen. There is no tendency to hæmorrhages from the stomach or intestinal tract."

Dr. Chartres stated to the Commission that "he thought that Sand-fly fever occurred at Bathurst; in fact, he considered that an attack of fever associated with severe headache from which he had suffered might have been due to that disease. Sandflies at certain seasons of the year were extremely numerous. He had not observed the occurrence of Dengue at Bathurst."

In a report by Drs. J. M. Dalziel and W. B. Johnson the following occurs:— Report on Yellow Fev Investigatio in Freetowi September, 1913, to March, 191 I.R., Vol. I pp. 541—5: (p. 554).

"No *Culicoides* or *Phlebotomus* have been observed by us during our six months, but they were not altogether absent from Bonthe, and they are stated to be abundant in some parts of the Protectorate."

Seven Days' Fever.

The nature of the fever thus named by Rogers is doubtful. By many it is regarded as Dengue.

Dr. J. W. Scott-Macfie's Report, quoted above, refers to this fever as follows:—

"Three cases (Nos. 7, 9, and 10), occurring in Europeans at Forcados and Burutu, have been provisionally diagnosed as seven days' fever. The symptoms were as follows:—The fever lasted for seven to nine days, and was saddlebacked in type; the pulse was relatively slow; the patients were prostrated, and suffered from severe pains in the back, and from headache. A rash, 'like rubella,' was observed in two of the cases. There was no albuminuria. The details of the cases, which occurred in 1909, are somewhat scanty; but in the absence L. 7. L. 9. L. 10.

of any mention of jaundice, hæmatemesis, catarrhal symptoms, sore throat, swellings of the joints, and malarial parasites, they may be regarded as suggestive of seven days' fever, or the saddleback type of dengue fever, which is considered by some authors to be the same disease."

Dr. Bailey, West African Medical Staff, who has been stationed chiefly in Southern Nigeria, stated to the Commission that—

"In 1909 he had had some cases of fever in Europeans which he had thought at the time might be seven-day fever, as described by Rogers. The grounds of his suspicion were that in two of the three cases there was a very marked pain in the back, and in all there was a saddleback temperature. There was no albuminuria when the tests of the urine were made, but there was a rash in two cases which he thought was not quite the same as Rogers'; the rash was very persistent in one case, lasting some time after convalescence. There was a slow pulse, but no itching of the hands. All three cases occurred within two months; one was fatal, but there was no post-mortem examination. That case had been in close contact with the others."

The following case, which occurred at Lokoja, in Northern Nigeria, on September 21st, 1913, in a European, aet. 30, was classified as "Possibly Seven Days' Fever" by the Commission.

"P. A. A., æt. 30, British. He had been travelling on the Benue river, visiting a sleeping sickness area.* Admitted to hospital, September 21st, 1913.

"Complains of pain in back and legs: Intense frontal headache and pains in the eyes. Face flushed: conjunctivæ injected. Skin dry. Pulse 96, resp. 18. Tongue thickly coated with white fur. No epigastric tenderness. No nausea or vomiting. Stools bilious. Nervous system depressed. Urine, Sp. gr. 1030. No albumen, blood or bile pigment No rash. Seven examinations of the blood for malaria parasites were negative.

"Sept. 24th. Leucocyte count:—

Leucocytes	17·2
Mononuclear	10·25
Polymorphonuclear	72·7

"Blood serum was negative to Widal: typhoid and paratyphoid *A* and *B*.

"During the illness the pulse varied from 86 to 60, the respirations from 24 to 16. There was a slight degree of diarrhœa.

"The temperature chart is annexed. The patient had no quinine from the date of admission up to September 30th.

* This patient was subsequently (December, 1914) found to be suffering from sleeping sickness.

"There was a small dark-coloured area on one of his legs, about the size of a threepenny piece, which rapidly increased to the size of a five-shilling piece, but it did not suppurate and was not tender; the swelling subsided.

"On Sept. 30th there was soreness of the naso-pharynx and a small ulcer appeared behind the left pillar of the fauces."

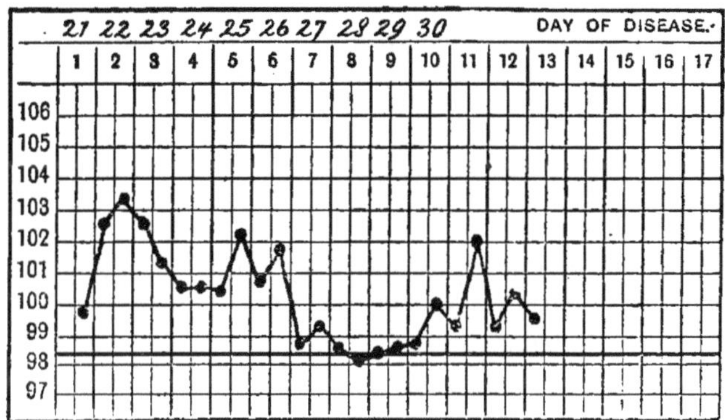

SECTION II.

TYPHOID AND PARATYPHOID FEVERS.

One case of typhoid at Sierra Leone was proved bacteriologically. The patient was a sailor on a German cruiser, and it is not certain that the disease was contracted on the Coast. Two cases with typhoid symptoms were observed amongst West African soldiers. Colonel Statham expresses the opinion that typhoid will be proved to exist amongst the West African natives.

Typhoid fever was certainly present in Freetown in 1884 (*vide* Second Report, p. 37). One of Colonel Statham's cases is classed as paratyphoid. The organism found closely resembled that isolated from a similar case, which occurred in December, 1912, but owing to difficulties of transport the culture flasks in both cases were contaminated, and it was not certain that the organism isolated was actually the cause of the condition, although clinically both cases presented the characters of a mild typhoid infection.

Dr. Butler also observed two cases of typhoid fever at Sierra Z. 6.*
Leone; in one case, which was fatal, the diagnosis was confirmed Z. 1.
on post-mortem examination; the second was proved by the agglutination reaction.

* For explanation of these numbers see footnote, page 12.

At Freetown, Sierra Leone, a male native, aet. 19, was admitted to hospital on September 1st, 1913, with pyrexia; diagnosed as Enteric Fever.

"Onset 25.8.13, sudden, with rigor and pain in back, but no headache; vomited once.

"Headache appeared on August 29th. No conjunctival injection; no flushing; no jaundice. Spleen enlarged. Tongue clean, inclined to be dry; no epigastric tenderness; no nausea or vomiting.

"Stools loose, pea-soup character, about 6 daily. Pulse 112-132, resp. 36.

"Dull, occasional delirium.

"Cloud of albumen in urine. No rash.

"Widal reaction positive to typhosus, negative to paratyphosus *A* or *B*. No malaria parasites on two examinations.

"Type of temperature: Remittent.

"Duration of pyrexia: 26 days.

"Termination: Recovery."

In the report on their investigation in Sierra Leone from September, 1913, to March, 1914 (*vide* I.R., Vol. II., pp. 541-578), by Drs. J. M. Dalziel and W. B. Johnson, it is stated (p. 549) that two cases proved to be *Enteric* with a positive Widal reaction for *B. typhosus*. In one of these cases the reaction was positive up to dilutions of 1/800, while negative except for group reactions in 1/20 dilutions, for *B. paratyphosus A.* and *B.*

Dr. J. W. Scott-Macfie in a report entitled "A Synopsis of Cases of Fever reported from Nigeria to the Medical Research Institute, Yaba, S. Nigeria, up to July 22nd, 1913," states under Typhoid Fever:—

"Eight cases have been reported that appeared to be typhoid fever. Seven (Nos. 11, 13, 28, 29, 30, 31 and 32) occurred in natives and one (No. 27) in a European. Two of the cases occurred at Burutu, one at Calabar, and five at Lokoja. One case (No. 32) terminated fatally.

"*European case.*—The one case in a European (No. 27) occurred at Calabar. The symptoms and the course of the disease presented a typical appearance, and the serum of the patient, which was kindly examined by the investigators at Sekondi, was reported as giving a positive Widal reaction for typhoid.

"*Native cases.*—Of the native cases, four (Nos. 28, 29, 30 and 31), all of which occurred at Lokoja, were typical of the disease. The fifth case from Lokoja (No. 32) was only diagnosed after death, on finding at the post-mortem examination numerous ulcers in the small intestine.

"The remaining two (Nos. 11 and 13) occurred at Burutu, and are at any rate suggestive of typhoid fever, complicated in the one case (No. 11) by febrile albuminuria, and in the other (No. 13) by otitis media."

Dr. H. A. Foy, in an interview with the Advisory Medical and Sanitary Committee for Tropical Africa, on 5th October, 1915, stated "that he had recently seen typhoid and paratyphoid and isolated the bacillus at Kano from a case of paratyphoid *A.*—a diagnosis confirmed by positive reaction from the blood test, and a culture of the bacillus isolated was sent to Lagos where it was verified as *B. paratyphosus A.* The case was that of a young European in the Political Department, who suffered from a low fever with diarrhœa, varying in intensity, for from fourteen to fifteen days, after which he got better and was allowed to get up, and later on to return to duty. In a week or ten days he had a relapse, and for fourteen days more he suffered from an illness of the same character as previously. It happened that Dr. Foy visited Kano shortly after this relapse to investigate an outbreak of dysentery in the prison. The Medical Officer in charge of the case asked him to look at it, and he took specimens of the blood, urine, and fæces, and made cultures from the latter. He saw none of the clinical symptoms."

The following cases are given as illustrating the frequency of continued fevers of a doubtful nature.

A case which occurred at Lokoja, in Northern Nigeria, on L. 29.
March 7th, 1913, was classified as "Possibly Typhoid":—

"Native: Hausa. W.A.F.F.

"Admitted 7th March, 1913.

"Duration of fever: 37 days.

"Character of fever: Remittent.

"Onset, with intense headache and depression; the latter continued until the headache was relieved.

"Tongue coated; no epigastric tenderness; no vomiting. One or two fluid stools daily, yellow in colour.

"No albumen in urine.

"Skin dry; no rash.

"Four examinations of blood were negative to malaria.

"Other cases of a similar nature were occurring in barracks."

The temperature chart shows a pyrexia of remittent type, ranging between 102° F. and 99° F. (105° F. on admission), a fall by lysis, and a nearly normal temperature about the 27th day; normal after the 37th day.

58. A case which occurred at Lokoja in July, 1913, was classified by the Commission as "Possibly Typhoid":-

"Negro. Aet. 19.

"Onset 7.7.13, with severe headache and pain in the splenic region. Temperature 101° F., pulse 100, resp. 24. Tongue white and furred; no epigastric tenderness; no nausea or vomiting; no jaundice. Two semi-solid motions daily.

"Depressed nervous condition; no rash.

"Urine contained albumen, blood and granular casts.

"No malaria parasites.

"Similar cases were occurring among his family or neighbours. No other details given.

"Type of fever: Irregular. Remittent.

"Duration of fever: 30 days.

"Defervescence by lysis."

The following case occurred at Lagos, on February 11th, 1911,
65. and was reported to the Commission by Dr. Craig (West African Medical Staff). It was diagnosed by them as ? Typhoid ? Paratyphoid.

"Male. Aet. 43.

"European.

"Onset 11th February, 1911. Result: Recovery.

"Symptoms: Vomiting and feeling of distension.

"Tongue furred.

"Slight epigastric tenderness.

"Vomiting during the first four days.

"Pulse 80, regular: mitral murmur.

"No albumen in urine.

"Rose spots or papules on abdomen.

"Widal twice negative to typhoid. Not tried for paratyphoid *A* or *B*."

Dr. Craig's diagnosis was:—

"A case of Enteric Fever, followed by a deep abscess after injection.

"Character of pyrexia: Remittent.

"Duration of fever: 10 days."

The following case which occurred at Burutu, in Southern Nigeria, on January 22nd, 1913, was classified as "Possibly Typhoid":— L. 11.

"Name: Abumselu.

"Race: Negro.

"Age: 30.

"Sex: Male.

"Occupation: Engineer.

"Date of admission to hospital: 22nd January, 1913.

"Date of discharge: 13th February, 1913.

"History.—Of three weeks' fever.

"Condition on admission:—Admitted *very prostrate*—wasted. Temperature 105° Fahr. Pulse 120. Eyes—no jaundice. No vomiting. Liver slightly enlarged and tender. Chest, some natural râles. Urine, no albumen; bilious appearance, but nitric acid test negative. Blood, negative.

"Course: 30th January.—Cloud of albumen appeared in urine and remained till 4th February.

"27th January.—Patient began complaining bitterly of burning pain in soles of feet. This symptom persisted after discharge. K.J.'s were present.

"The fever took a long time to wear out; finally after nearly three weeks the temperature became sub-normal and of moderate excursion and convalescence started.

"The case completed showed a fever *not malaria*, characterized by *great prostration*, albumen in urine, no jaundice or vomiting, pulse rate not helpful, no parasites in blood, a slow convalescence with no relapse."

The following case, which occurred at Burutu, S. Nigeria, on April 8, 1913, was classified as "Possibly Paratyphoid." It is noted that there were "other similar cases at Burutu." L 13.

"Name: James II.

"Race: Negro.

"Age: 29.

"Sex: Male.

"Occupation: Labourer.

"Date of admission to hospital: 8th April, 1913.

"Date of discharge: 18th April, 1913.

"History.—Admitted so deaf as to be useless for any history.

"Condition on admission.—Temperature, 103·4° Fahr. Pulse, 124. Tongue, coated with fur. Spleen, enlarged two fingers below ribs. Albuminuria marked. Deafness ceased on 25th April.

"Case completed shows a fever, not malarial, characterized by: Albuminuria. Slow pulse. White fur on tongue. Deafness."

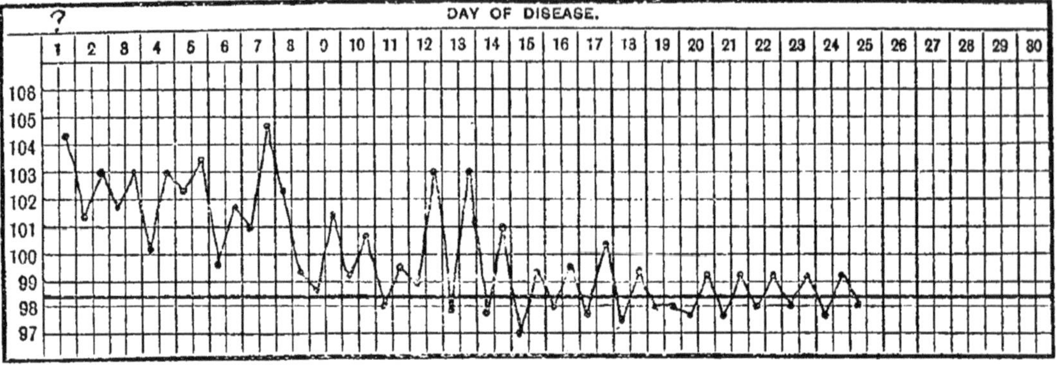

SECTION III.

UNDULANT FEVER. PARA-UNDULANT FEVER.

rk done at etown n May 1st 'eptember h, 1913; . Vol. II., 389–416 393).

ort of a es of 800 dical exias, etc. . Vol. II., 353–386 383).

One case of "possibly undulant fever" is referred to by Dr. Butler (p. 393).

It was reported from Daru by Dr. Mayhew (West African Medical Staff) on a card.

Colonel Statham observes (p. 383): "*Undulant Fever.*—Though no case has yet been found where the blood reacted with the *Micrococcus melitensis* (and several have been tried), yet as goats abound in Freetown and the milk is sometimes drunk by natives, I think Undulant Fever may be present in Sierra Leone."

In the report by Drs. H. Sinclair Coghill and H. M. Hänschell, "On Work at Sekondi from 1st October, 1913, to 30th April, 1914" (*vide* I.R., Vol. II., p., 714), it is stated that "Serum from two cases —one European, one native—was sent by Dr. W. J. Bruce from Abosso with details of the cases. The serum in both cases agglutinated *Micrococcus melitensis* in dilution of 1/80—complete in 3 hours. No clumping was obtained with control bacteria, *e.g.*, *B. typhosus* and *B. paratyphosus.* With normal control serum the bouillon culture of *M. melitensis* gave partial clumping up to 1/20 dilution only."

SECTION IV.

TYPHUS. ROCKY-MOUNTAIN FEVER. DOUBLE CONTINUED FEVER. CEREBRO-SPINAL FEVER.

No example of any one of these fevers has been reported to the Commission as occurring during the three years covered by their investigations.*

The nature of bilious remittent fever in its various forms is fully considered in Part III. sections.

SECTION V.

CONCLUSIONS.

From the evidence given above, the Commission are of opinion that the following fevers have been met with in the West African Colonies, viz.:—Pappataci Fever, Typhoid and Paratyphoid Fevers, and (possibly) Undulant Fever and Seven Days' Fever. As regards Dengue, its presence there cannot be held to have been proved. The evidence does not suggest that any one of the fevers named is widely prevalent.

* Dr. A. E. Horn reported in 1908 on an Investigation of two Outbreaks of Cerebro-Spinal Fever in the Northern Territories of the Gold Coast in 1906 and 1907-8. (Report published by the Government Printer, Accra). In the Report he refers to a "severe epidemic in Northern Nigeria" in 1905, and says that serious outbreaks have occurred in the latter Dependency "at intervals during the last fifty years."

PART III.

YELLOW FEVER.

SYNOPSIS.

SECTION I.

INTRODUCTORY.

The Historical Retrospect of the occurrence of Yellow Fever in the Dependencies, both British and foreign, on the West Coast of Africa, which forms the greater part of the Second Report of the Commission, was undertaken in order to determine whether Yellow Fever was then present on that Coast, and if so, whether it had been there for a very long period.

These questions may now be regarded as settled. If in this Report the same ground is traversed to some extent, it is with a different object.

We are now specially concerned to discover, if possible, what were the factors which led to the occurrence of epidemics and sporadic cases of that disease during the period under review; what influence the slave trade in its various phases had upon the incidence of the disease; what places may be considered to have been endemic foci where its presence was continuous, and how they ceased to possess that character.

The types of Yellow Fever met with in natives and Europeans, the symptomatology, diagnosis, pathological anatomy and cytology of that disease, and other questions of importance connected therewith, are considered in detail in this part of the report, and it is hoped that the study which has been given to these points has brought to light some facts which may help to solve the many problems which still surround the subject of the endemic and epidemic prevalence of Yellow Fever on the West Coast of Africa.

SECTION II.

THE NOMENCLATURE OF VARIOUS FORMS OF FEVER.

The difficulty which is referred to in the previous report, of deciding when we are certainly dealing with Yellow Fever, is no doubt considerable, but it diminishes to some extent as one's acquaintance with the terms used by the writers on the subject increases.

All the writers believed that the types of fever common on the Coast were variants from a single stock, and that the less severe types could under certain conditions be transformed into those of a graver character.

When the fever is described as "intermittent," we can hardly be wrong in concluding that malaria is to be understood; when again, at the other end of the scale, the terms "malignant," "pernicious remittent," "pernicious malignant," "the severe form of typho-malarial or yellow fever" are employed, there can be little doubt that the disease may have been Yellow Fever, but it may also have been Malaria of the pernicious æstivo-autumnal type. The real difficulty arises over the meaning to be attached to the terms "remittent fever" and "bilious remittent fever." This point is discussed in detail in a later section of the Report. The latter term was, no *Vide* p. 16 doubt, frequently used to describe attacks of Yellow Fever, some of which proved fatal, whilst others ended in recovery, but it was also applied to cases which, with an equal degree of certainty, we may conclude to have been due to Malaria. An example of this will be found on page 15 of the Second Report, in the following extract from the Annual Report from the Gold Coast for 1849:—

> "Nineteen cases of seasoning or remittent fever occurred amongst newly arrived Europeans. Of these, six, who received no medical attendance, died, and thirteen, who were treated with large doses of quinine, all recovered. In the most obstinate cases the fever was checked within twenty-four hours."

In Appendix I. of this Report an interesting observation by Dr. Chacin Itriago, of Venezuela, will be found on the beneficial effect of intramuscular injections of quinine on the course of cases of Yellow Fever in the subjects of Malaria.

A consideration of the following extracts from the "Annual Medical Report for 1869 on the troops stationed at Sierra Leone" renders it difficult to avoid the conclusion that the author, Staff-Surgeon Gore, regarded "Remittent Fever" as a manifestation of the presence of a poison which, according to its degree of virulence, produced either Remittent Fever or Yellow Fever:—

> "Two varieties of these [epidemic visitations] have visited the Colony of Sierra Leone at uncertain intervals of time. The first, such as *yellow fever* or *malignant remittent*, is principally confined to

the Europeans, whereas the second class, such as variola, varicella, dengue or broken bone fever and dysentery, have been almost altogether felt in their severity by the native."

"The earlier years of Colonial existence, especially 1807, 1809, 1812, 1815 and 1819, appear to have been ones of extreme unhealthiness from the severity of the *endemic remittent*, but this fever has always had up to the present time seasons of exacerbations, during some years assuming a very mild form, at others a most severe, the mortality increasing with the latter. It also has not infrequently occurred that a prevalence of severe remittent was a warning of the approach of its more deadly sister, *or extensively prevailed whilst the latter was epidemic.*"

"On the previous December* (1822) an isolated case of malignant fever, with coffee ground vomit, ended fatally. The individual had come from on board a ship in harbour, timber vessels, the crews of which at the time were very unhealthy, several having died in hospital from the *endemic remittent.*"

"In 1825 a large body of white troops arrived at Sierra Leone: the sickness and mortality amongst them was so great as to approach the character of an epidemic. During the second quarter of the year *remittent fever* of a virulent and fatal form set in. Out of 902 attacked, 263 succumbed to the disease, which only differed from yellow fever in having no coffee ground vomit at its termination. In several the occurrence of yellow suffusion and bleeding from the gums took place a few hours before dissolution."

"In February and May, 1837, epidemic yellow fever again broke out in Sierra Leone. On this, as on other similar occasions, the epidemic outbreak was not sudden, but was preceded, so far back as the month of January, by several suspicious cases of the *ordinary endemic remittent* or country fever. These cases were of great severity, two of them proving fatal."

"Of this epidemic it is related that 'it greatly ceased by almost imperceptible and indefinable lines, *merging into the ordinary endemic remittent*, the cases occurring at its termination nearly all recovering.'"

"During July, August and September of 1839 a severe form of *remittent fever* caused six deaths in Tower Hill Barracks. With one exception, every officer belonging to the Royal African Corps suffered in greater or less degree; seven naval officers and thirteen seamen also died of the disease."

"In 1845 *remittent fever* prevailed to a great extent amongst the squadron at Sierra Leone, causing several deaths: one, occurring in the quarter ending September 30th, was an unequivocal case of *malignant remittent or yellow fever*, with coffee ground vomit; two other cases also occurred in civil practice."

"The '*Eclair*' left the Colony in this year on July 23rd; upwards of 60 of the crew perished during the voyage from yellow fever."

* "The first really severe epidemic of yellow fever" is said to have occurred in 1823.

These extracts are sufficient to prove that the author of this Report considered that the fevers variously named therein were manifestations of one and the same disease, and that it was a question of degree and not of kind.

SECTION III.

DIFFERENT PERIODS ON THE COAST.

In considering the prevalence of Yellow Fever on the West Coast of Africa it will be convenient to divide the years under review into the following periods:—

(*a*) The periods of unrestricted slave trade and of maritime blockade up to the date of the more or less complete suppression of the slave trade, about the year 1850.

(*b*) From the abolition of the slave trade (circ. 1850) to 1900.

(*c*) From 1900 to the date of the appointment of the Commission in January, 1913.

(*d*) From January, 1913, to December, 1915.

SECTION IV.

THE PERIODS OF UNRESTRICTED SLAVE TRADE AND OF MARITIME BLOCKADE UP TO THE DATE OF THE MORE OR LESS COMPLETE SUPPRESSION OF THE SLAVE TRADE, ABOUT THE YEAR 1850.

In attempting to estimate the influence of the slave trade upon the spread of Yellow Fever, and on the occurrence of epidemics of that disease in the Dependencies of the West Coast of Africa, it is important to bear in mind that this traffic was essentially an export trade. The slaves were obtained from the interior and were shipped for transmission to the West Indies and elsewhere.

The following extracts are from "the Annual Report to accompany the return of sick and wounded of the troops stationed at

Sierra Leone for the year ending 31st December, 1869," by Staff-Surgeon Albert A. Gore, M.D., Principal Medical Officer:—

"In 1434 Antonio Gonzales shipped slaves from Western Africa, and is said to have visited Sierra Leone in 1441."

"Sir John Hawkins landed at Sierra Leone 8th May, 1562, returning to England 3rd September, 1563. He subsequently made three voyages to Africa, bought slaves and sold them to the Spanish settlements in America."

"In 1588 Queen Elizabeth was induced to grant patents for carrying on the slave trade from the North of the Senegal to 100 leagues below Sierra Leone."

"During 1697 the slave trade was sanctioned by the English Parliament."

"In 1752 an Act of Parliament (23 Geo. II., Cap. 31) was passed, making the slave trade free to all His Majesty's subjects, provided a sufficient number of negroes were supplied at a reasonable rate. By this Act the settlements upon the West Coast were vested in the company of African merchants."

"In 1764 this Act was repealed, the officer and servants on the coast being prohibited from exporting negroes on their own account."

"In 1787 Sierra Leone passed from the hands of the Portuguese into those of the English, who colonised it by the importation of 342 settlers from England."

"On the 1st July, 1791, the Sierra Leone Company was established on the condition of their not dealing in or employing slaves."

"Sixteen vessels arrived at Sierra Leone in 1792, having on board 1,131 Nova Scotians. The original intent was to make the Colony a home for free Africans, hoping thereby to raise Colonial produce without slave labour. Of the 100 Europeans who composed the first settlement, 57 died during the first rainy season; 800 blacks were also attacked with fever."

After various fruitless efforts in Parliament from 1792 to 1806, a Bill was passed in the latter year to put an end to the British slave trade for foreign supply, and to forbid the importation of slaves into the Colonies won by the British arms in the course of the war.

In 1807 a Bill was passed for the abolition of the slave trade.

This Act was habitually violated, and in 1811 an Act was passed declaring the traffic in slaves to be a felony punishable with transportation. This Act proved effective and brought the trade to an end, so far as the British dominions were concerned.

In 1826 a convention was entered into between Great Britain and Brazil, but it was habitually violated in spite of the English cruisers.

By the connivance of the local administrative authorities 54,000 Africans were annually exported.

In 1850 the trade is said to have been decisively put down.

Dr. Alexander Bryson, a naval surgeon, was appointed,* probably in 1845, by the Lords' Commissioners of the Admiralty "to go over the whole of the returns received into the Admiralty since the year 1820, and to embody in a report the greatest amount of information regarding the diseases contracted on the African Station, the localities most injurious to health, the precautions which might be taken to avert or diminish fever, and the mode of treatment regarded most effectual; embracing also the diseases most prevalent amongst the captured slaves." The report covers the period from 1820-1845.

Report on the Climate and Principal Diseases of the African Station by Alexander Bryson, M.D., Surgeon, R.N., 1847.

The report commences thus:—

> "During the first ten years of the period included in this report (*i.e.*, 1820-9) the traffic in slaves was vigorously prosecuted under the flags of several nations on different parts of the coast from the Gambia on the north to Benguela on the south of the equator, while from certain anomalous clauses in the treaties then in existence, as the right of capture did not extend to vessels sailing to the south of the line under Brazilian colours, *where for the sake of security they were generally assumed*, the operations of the British cruisers were principally although not entirely confined to the northern latitudes between the parallel of Cape Verd and the equator."

The report of Dr. Bryson necessarily deals chiefly with "Fever," but the author recognised only remittent and intermittent fever of various grades of severity, and he gives no clinical descriptions by which the various types of fever might be differentiated. Yellow Fever is not mentioned, and in the section of the report devoted to the diseases most prevalent amongst the captured slaves, that disease does not find a place.

---

* The report is dated 1847.

> "The diseases from which negro slaves suffer most severely on board the vessels destined for their transportation are dysentery, fever, small-pox, ophthalmia and diarrhœa." (p. 255.)

Craw-craw, guinea worm and yaws are also described as being very prevalent amongst the slaves.

The following extracts deal with the diseases prevalent amongst the sailors of ships of the Navy engaged in the suppression of the slave trade and particularly with Sierra Leone (p. 7):—

n. p. 7.

> "Sierra Leone, being by far the most important of our settlements * * * * * * has long been one of the principal resorts of the squadron * * * * * *. Spanish and Brazilian vessels captured by the squadron are also sent to Sierra Leone for adjudication in the Court of mixed Commission, each with a prize crew on board consisting of from ten to twenty white men and a few blacks * * * * * *."
>
> "Whether this Colony is more detrimental to the European constitution than other localities of the Coast it would be difficult to determine, but that a far greater proportional amount of disease is contracted here by the naval force than upon any other part of the station is clearly evident, at least since Fernando Po has been abandoned. * * * * * * native Africans * * * * * * are happily, though natives of a different part of the continent, exempt from the diseases which prove so fatal to Europeans." (p. 7.)
>
> "It appears, however, that the officers and men who navigate prize vessels to Sierra Leone suffer most severely. They generally arrive worn out by excessive labour, broken rest and exposure by night and day upon the deck of a small vessel, probably crowded with slaves in a loathsome state of misery and disease." (p. 9.)
>
> "They take up their quarters in a building in the town * * * * * * denominated 'the Barn.' Many, while they still inhabit the Barn, are seized with fever, and are taken to the military hospital; others escape for a time, and apparently enjoy good health until they embark either in their own vessel or some other, which may in the meantime opportunely arrive; but in either case it generally happens that *they are attacked with the disease within two weeks from the date of joining.* Few entirely escape the danger of this ordeal, even if they be of the most orderly and temperate habits." (p. 9.)

The duration of the period of freedom from disease—two weeks from the date of joining—does not point to Yellow Fever infection occurring whilst on board the slave ship.

The Extent of the Slave Trade.

The extent of the traffic in slaves is seen from the following tabular statement* contained in the "Report of the Lords of the

* Evidence of Mr. Norris. Part II.

Committee of Council appointed 11th February, 1788, for the consideration of all matters relating to trade and foreign relations, particularly concerning the present state of the trade to Africa and particularly the trade in slaves."

"The whole of the very extensive coast of Negroland supplies the following numbers yearly:—

Gambia	700
Isles de Los and the adjacent rivers	1,500
From Sierra Leone to Cape Mount	2,000
Cape Mount to Cape Palmas	3,000
Cape Palmas to Cape Appollonia	1,000
The Gold Coast	10,000
Quilta and Popoe	1,000
Wydah	4,500
Porta Nova Eppee and Kidagry	3,500
Lagos and Benin	3,500
Bonny and New Calabar	14,500
Old Calabar and Cameroons	7,000
Gabon and Cape Lopez	500
Loango Melimba and Cahenda	13,500
Majumba Ambies and Miasonla	1,000
Loango St. Paul's and Benguilla	7,000
	74,200

Of these the British purchase about ...	38,000
" " " French " " ...	20,000
" " " Dutch " " ...	4,000
" " " Danes " " ...	2,000
" " " Portuguese " " ...	10,000
	74,000

The Slave Trade in Relation to Yellow Fever.

The "Virginia Medical Monthly" for April, 1875, contains an article entitled "Researches on the relations of the African Slave Trade in the West Indies and Tropical America to Yellow Fever," by Joseph Jones, M.D., Professor of Chemistry and Clinical Medicine in the Medical Department of the University of Louisiana.

In a letter to a member of the Commission the author is described, by one well able to judge, as "a remarkable man, born out of due time and place."

The following extracts are from this article:—

"If the history of yellow fever in the Western hemisphere be considered in a general way, it will be found that the accounts and dates of its origin vary with the extent and character of the information of the writers in different localities and in different nationalities. Thus, some have referred the origin of the disease to the crowded African slavers, with their freights of suffering and enslaved humanity.

"Within a few years after the discovery of the West India Islands by the Spaniards the mild and unsuspecting natives had, for the greater part, perished. Millions of them were swept from the face of the earth by reason of the cruelty and avarice of desperate, immoral and murderous adventurers from the West."

"When the Spaniards found how rapidly the aboriginal population of the West India Islands perished under the system of forced labour, and beneath the tyranny of their rule, the expedient of introducing negro slaves from Africa was resorted to. The example of the Spaniards was soon followed by the Portuguese, Dutch, French and English: companies for the traffic were formed, monopolies granted. Before the close of the sixteenth century the African slave-trade was carried on by natives of nearly all the maritime States of Europe, and, in after times, with great vigour by the United States of America, the great majority of the 'slavers' from this country being fitted out, equipped, provisioned and manned in the ports of the Northern and New England States. For three centuries the most civilised of the European nations prosecuted a sanguinary traffic in human beings on the coast of Western Africa, dragged into bondage upwards of 25,000,000 of her unfortunate children.

"The following observations embrace the most important facts developed by our researches, established with the design of determining the connection of yellow fever with the African slave-trade.

"In the year 1442, while the Portuguese* were exploring the coasts of Africa, Anthony Gonsalez, who, two years before, had seized some Moors near Cape Bojardi, was, by Prince Henry, ordered to carry his prisoners back to Africa. He landed them at Rio del Oro, and received from the Moors in exchange ten blacks and a quantity of gold dust, with which he returned to Lisbon. The success of Gonsalez not only awakened the admiration, but stimulated the avarice of his countrymen, who, in the course of a few succeeding years, fitted out no less than thirty-seven ships in pursuit of the same traffic. In 1481 the Portuguese built a fort on the Gold Coast, another some time afterwards on the Island of Arguin, and a third at Loango Saint Paul's, on the coast of Angola: and the King of Portugal took the title of Lord of

* "Hist. Brit. Colonies: West Indies." Edwards. Vol. II, pp. 239—262.

Guinea. So rapid, however, was the decrease of the unfortunate natives as to induce the Court of Spain, a few years afterwards, to revoke the orders issued by Oriando, and to authorise by royal authority the introduction of African slaves from the Portuguese settlements on the coasts of Guinea. In the year 1517 Emperor Charles V. granted a patent to certain persons for the exclusive supply of 4,000 negroes annually to the islands of Hispaniola, Cuba, Jamaica and Puerto Rico. This patent having been supplied to some Genoese merchants, the supply of negroes to the Spanish American plantations became from that time an established and regular branch of commerce.

" In 1637, after the English had begun their settlement of plantations in the West Indies, negroes were in such demand as to induce the formation of a new company for the prosecution of the African slave-trade: and King Charles I. granted to sundry merchants the exclusive right to enjoy the sole trade to the coast of Guinea, between Cape Blanco and the Cape of Good Hope, together with the isles adjacent, for thirty-one years."

" What has been quoted is sufficient to demonstrate that the Portuguese established the slave trade before the discovery of America by Columbus; that as early as 1502 the Spaniards began to employ negroes in the mines of Hispaniola; and that a regular traffie in slaves had been established so early as the year 1564 by several nations, as the Portuguese, Spaniards, French and English."

" Of the diseases developed amongst these miserable people, whilst confined in the slave marts of the African coast, and upon the crowded and filthy slavers during their horrible passage across the Atlantic we have only imperfect accounts. *In 1669 a fatal epidemic fever prevailed in St. Domingo, and its introduction was ascribed to slave ships from the coast of Africa, and the local authorities passed ordinances to prevent the introduction of contagious and malignant fevers by means of slaves.* (*Moreau de Jonnes, p.* 58-59.)"

" We extract the following observations upon the conduct of the slave trade and the diseases of the negroes in the West India islands, from the valuable work of Bryan Edwards. (Hist. West Indies, Vol. II., p. 328, 1791):—

" In sickness the invalids are immediately removed to the captain's cabin, or to a hospital built near the forecastle, and treated with all the care, both in regard to medicine and food, that circumstances will admit; and when, fortunately for the negroes, the ship touches at any place in her voyage, as frequently happens, any refreshment that the country affords, as cocoa-nuts, oranges, limes and other fruits, with vegetables of all sorts, are distributed among them: and refreshments of the same kind are freely allowed them at the place of their destination, between the days of arrival and sail."

" At the ports of Montego Bay, in Jamaica, the negroes imported between the 18th day of November, 1789, and the 15th of July, 1791, were 9,993, in 38 ships; the mortality at sea, exclusive of the loss of 54 negroes in a mutiny on the coast, was 746, which is somewhat under 7 per cent. of the whole number of slaves. This, though much less,

I believe, than the average loss which happened before the regulating law took place, is, I admit, sufficiently great: and had it prevailed in any degree equally on the several ships concerned might, perhaps, have been considered as a fair estimate of the general mortality consequent on the trade, notwithstanding the peculiarities and provisions of the regulating act. On examining the list, I find that eight of the thirty-eight ships were entitled to, and actually received, the full premium; two others received the half premium, and one other (a schooner that sailed from Jamaica to the coast before the Act took place) returned without the loss of a single negro. Of the 746 deaths, no less than 328 occurred in four ships only, all of which, with five other vessels, comprehending the whole number of ships in which three-fifths of the mortality occurred, came from the same part of the coast, the Bight of Benin: a circumstance that gives room to conclude (as was undoubtedly the fact) that the negroes from that part of the country brought disease and contagion with them from the land: *an epidemic fever and flux generally prevailing on the low marshy shores of Bonny during the autumnal months, which sometimes proves even more destructive on shore than at sea.*" (pp. 332-333.)

"It is difficult to determine from this description whether the epidemic contagious fever and flux, here alluded to as prevailing on the low marshy shores of the Bonny Rivers, attacked the natives, or only those Europeans engaged in the slave trade. It is well established that the negroes are not, as a general rule, subject to Yellow Fever either upon the coast of Africa or in the tropical regions. They have suffered, however, to a certain extent from this disease in some epidemics, and it is possible that they may have suffered from this fever when subjected to the foul atmosphere of the slaver. It appeared in evidence before the House of Commons that before the passage of the regulating Act, a ship of 240 tons would frequently be crowded with no less than 520 slaves, which was but allowing ten inches of room to each individual. The consequence of this barbârous avarice was ofttimes a loss of 15 per cent. in the voyage and 4½ per cent. more in the harbours of the West Indies. previous to the sale, from diseases contracted at sea."

"Bryan Edwards makes no mention of Yellow Fever amongst the diseases of the negroes in the West Indies, thus he says:—

"Among the diseases which negroes bring with them from Africa, the most loathsome are the *cacaba* and the *yaws*: and it is difficult to say which is the worst." (Hist. West Indies, Vol. II., p. 352.)

"The testimony of Abbé Raynal in his "*Philosophical and Political History of the Europeans in the East and West Indies,*" with reference to the diseases of the negroes in the West Indies, corresponds with that of Edwards.

"Thus he says that the African slaves in the West Indies 'are particularly subject to two diseases, the yaws and that complaint that affects their stomach.'"

"M. Dalzille, in his valuable and elaborate work, '*Observations sur Maladies des Nègres,*' refers the diseases of the Europeans in the

West Indies chiefly to the effects of heat and the stagnant marshes, and associates their production with the causes which favour the development and multiplication of animalculæ. In his observations upon the fevers of the negroes of the West Indies and more especially of St. Dominique, contained chiefly in Chap. I. of Vol. I., under the head of *fievres putrides*, describes the various forms of *malarial paroxysmal fever*, and fails to mention Yellow Fever.

"Dr. William Hillary, in his '*Treatise on such Diseases as are most frequent in or are peculiar to the West Indies or the Torrid Zone*,' whilst recording accurate descriptions of these diseases as the yaws and leprosy, peculiar to the negroes, makes no allusion to the prevalence of Yellow Fever amongst them, nor to the importation of this disease from Africa. Thus in the chapter on '*The Putrid Bilious Fever, commonly called the Yellow Fever*,' he says that :—

"From the best and most authentic accounts that I can obtain, as also from the nature and symptoms of the disease, it appears to be a fever that is indigenous to the West India Islands and the continent of America, which is situated between or near the tropics, and most probably to all other countries within the torrid zone."

"Dr. Benjamin Rush, who edited the works of Dr Hillary, in commenting upon the preceding statement, observes :—

"We have here a testimony against the non-contagiousness of the yellow fever by an eminent physician, who resided many years in one of those islands from which the disease has been said to be exported. It is probable, in the few cases in which the fever was said to be contagious, there was a mixture of the jail or ship fever with it : or the yellow fever may have been so protracted as to generate that matter which has been called 'contagion of excretion.' "

"The testimony of Dr. Hillary is of importance, especially as he has given one of the most accurate descriptions of Yellow Fever extant.

"Dr. Lind, in his treatise on the Jail Distemper, says, with reference to the diseases of the slave-ships :—

"The poor wretches are crowded together below the deck as close as they possibly can be, with only a small separation between the men and women. Every night they are shut up under close hutches, in a sultry climate, barred down with iron to prevent an insurrection : and though some have been suffocated by this close confinement in foul air, though they are subject to the flux, and suffer from a change of climate, yet an infection is scarcely known among them : or if an *accidental* fever, occurring from the change of climate, should become infectious, it is generally much more mild than in the opposite situation." ("On Preserving the Health of Seamen," Sec. Ed., p. 317-318.)

"Dr. Thomas Trotter, who was himself surgeon to a slave ship, says :—

"The situation of the African negroes confined during the middle passage, in the slave rooms of a Guineaman, has been mentioned by

Dr. Lind. The confinement of so many irrational creatures in a small space deservedly attracted the animadversions of a physician investigating the sources and progress of contagion. *But contagious fevers, we find, are not their diseases.* We can well believe that if the negroes were clothed that filth and uncleanness might generate infection: the excessive quantity of perishable matter emitted from the surface in a high degree of heat would soon accumulate, and adhering to linen or woollen cloths might at least propagate forms of disease. But the matter being daily washed from their skins, and the rooms kept clean, nothing offensive or of an animal origin is allowed to undergo the final decomposition, which it would do in nasty and unventilated clothing. Thus also the poor inhabitants of warm countries are free from the diseases of those in colder regions." ("Medicina Nautica: An Essay on the Diseases of Seamen," Second Edition, Vol. I., p. 184.)

"Dr. Garden, in a letter to Rev. Stephen Hayes, D.D., dated Charlestown, South Carolina, March 24th, 1756, after mentioning the Guinea slave-ships arriving there, adds:—

"I have often gone to visit these vessels on their first arrival, in order to make a report of their state of health to the Governor and Council: but I never yet was on board one that did not smell most offensive and noisesome: what from filth, putrid air, putrid dysenteries (which is their common disorder), it is a wonder that any escape with life." ("Hale's Treatise on Ventilators," Second Part, p. 95.)

"Dr. Edward Nathaniel Bancroft gives the most decided testimony against the origin of Yellow Fever in the African slaves. Thus he observes:—

"Dr. Lind, influenced as he was by the commonly received opinions, mentions an infection (meaning a fever) as being scarcely known in the slave-ships, instead of asserting, as he might have done with truth, that it is *never known;* for, after very extensive inquiries, I am fully convinced that fever of any kind rarely occurs on board these vessels, and *contagious fever* never: though great mortality has frequently happened from other disease, and more especially from dysentery." ("Essay on Yellow Fever," London, 1811, p. 128.)

"We conclude, therefore, from the preceding researches, *that Yellow Fever is not a disease of the African race, in tropical climates, and that the origin and propagation of the disease in Insular and Central America cannot be traced to the African slave-trade.*"

The researches of Dr. Jones do not lend much support to the view that the West African slave-trade was responsible to any considerable degree for the transmission of Yellow Fever, at any rate across the Atlantic. It is of interest to note, however, that in the only instance mentioned in which Yellow Fever may have been the disease which caused a high mortality on board the slave ships, the slaves had come from the Bight of Benin, which is precisely the part of the coast most likely to have been infected.

It will be remembered that in the Second Report, p. 89, extracts were given from the journal of the "*Bloodhound*," 1861 and 1862, by Mr. W. J. Eames, Assistant Surgeon in charge, from which it is clear that at that date "the rivers" were an infected area. "*The rivers seem to have suffered in more than an ordinary degree, the River Bonny in particular. The epidemic made its appearance in March, 1862, and raged with unabated violence for three months; out of 160 white inhabitants 130 died in that time. It was equally fatal amongst the natives.*"

Again in 1862 and 1863 "the rivers" are mentioned in the Journal.

> "*Arriving off the River Benin* on the night of the 3rd August we came to an anchor and remained there twenty-three days. It is much to be regretted that no medical man was in the river whose opinion on the nature of this disease which had made such havoc amongst the residents could be depended upon, but from a statement made to me by a resident there, a Mr. Henry, who had studied medicine, I have no doubt the disease was *the same that had depopulated all the other rivers in the Bights—Yellow Fever.*"

It does not of course follow that because Yellow Fever prevailed extensively in "the rivers" in 1862, it was there in 1791, but it is not in the nature of this disease, when firmly established, to lose its hold entirely, if all the surrounding conditions remain unchanged.

We have quoted at length from Dr. Jones's paper as its author was eminently qualified to deal with the question which he discusses, and had obviously studied the literature of the subject with care.

His general conclusions as to the nature of the diseases prevalent on the slave ships are partly borne out by the evidence of surgeons on slave ships given before the Committee of Council and the Committee of the House of Commons in 1789. Thus Surgeon Isaac Wilson states that in a voyage on a slaver of 370 tons "flux prevailed," and out of 602 slaves carried 155 died of that disease, "the slaves had no other very fatal disorder."

Dr. Falconbridge (House of Commons Committee), however, states that the most prevalent disorders were "fevers and dysenteries," but does not mention Yellow Fever.

As bearing upon the question of the liability to disease of the European crews of the slave ships the evidence of the Reverend Mr. Clarkson before the Lords Committee may be quoted. It contains an account of the muster rolls of 88 slave vessels that returned to

Liverpool in 1786, and up to the month of September, 1787, of which the following is a summary :—

			Similarly ot 24 Bristol ships.
Numbers of original crews which sailed from England or were taken in at Africa	3,170	...	910
Of these there returned to England ...	1,428	...	455
Died or were lost	642	...	216
Discharged on voyage either in Africa or the West Indies, or deserted ...	1,100	...	239

Other figures are given by the witness, who was one of the leaders of the Anti-slavery party, to show that the mortality amongst the crews of vessels engaged in other trades was far less than that on the slave ships; but he does not attempt to prove that the very high rate of mortality was due to any particular disease.

As bearing on the mortality amongst Europeans resident on the West Coast of Africa at and about the same date, the following figures, which are given in a return to the Lords Committee (1788), are of interest.

The return is headed thus :—

> "An account of the number of persons in a civil and military capacity who have been admitted into the service of the Company of Merchants trading to Africa since the year 1751, when the forts and settlements were surrendered by the Royal African Company to the Committee by Act of 23 of George the Second, together with the number of such persons who died the first year after their arrival in Africa or at any future period, and of those who quitted the service and took their discharges in Africa or returned to Europe."

1751 to 1788.

	Died in 1st year.	Died subsequently in Africa.	Total Deaths.	Took Discharge.
Civilians, 352 ...	94	320	653	369
Soldiers, 728 ...	239			

The above figures give a mortality in the first year of 30·8 per cent., and a total mortality of 60·4 per cent., the inference being that if this enormous death rate was due to Malaria that disease was then much more often fatal than it now is in Africa, or that other diseases, and amongst them possibly Yellow Fever, were partly responsible for the large number of deaths.

CONCLUSION.

We fear that we cannot claim that our own study of the literature of the subject has been more successful than that of Dr. Jones in throwing light upon the connection between the slave trade and the spread of Yellow Fever beyond Africa; probably there was little or no connection between them.

SECTION V.

FROM THE ABOLITION OF THE SLAVE TRADE (CIRC. 1850) TO 1900.

The Second Report of the Commission contains an account of what is known as regards the incidence of Yellow Fever during these years.

It would not, in the opinion of the Commission, serve any useful purpose to repeat in this section all that is there stated under the various Dependencies; any one who is interested in the subject can readily obtain an impression of the state of affairs, as regards Yellow Fever, on the coast as a whole during these years, from the descriptions given under each Dependency.

Moreover, this period includes the year 1862, of which a very complete and detailed account is given in the Second Report, *vide* p. 83. It may be remembered that this year was selected for such treatment, as it was the year during which the disease prevailed most extensively upon the coast.

SECTION VI.

FROM 1900 TO THE DATE OF THE APPOINTMENT OF THE COMMISSION IN JANUARY, 1913.

During the first ten years of this period the existence of Yellow Fever in the British Dependencies on the West Coast was barely recognised, and any Medical Officer who ventured upon such a diagnosis might possibly have found that his official superiors regarded him as an alarmist, and would be better pleased if, in future, such cases were returned either as "Malaria" or "Bilious Remittent Fever."

We have, however, already seen that the events which happened in 1910 rendered this attitude no longer possible.

The Second Report (*vide* p. 108) contains a general survey of the position as regards Yellow Fever on the West Coast of Africa immediately preceding and at the time of the first outbreak in May, 1910, at Freetown, and it is there shown that in 1910 the disease was present at various places distributed over a very wide area in West Africa.

The epidemics of 1910 at Freetown, at Seccondee and at Lagos; of 1911 at Accra and at Bathurst; of 1912 at various places on the Gold Coast, have been already described and analysed in the Second Report of the Commission, and it is unnecessary to traverse again the ground therein covered.

We shall therefore in this section deal chiefly with the earlier years of the period under review and only refer to the epidemics just mentioned in order to bring out points of importance not already dealt with.

The Commission adopted the following system in classifying suspected cases. After a careful examination of the whole of the available evidence the cases were placed in one of the following four classes:—

Yellow Fever.
Probable Yellow Fever.
Possible Yellow Fever.
Negative (where the evidence was insufficient for classification or some other disease was indicated).

In any instance in which there was a difference of opinion among the members of the Commission as to the classification this fact is stated.

This classification has one very great advantage, in as much as it approaches as nearly as possible to certainty, when a confident opinion is expressed, *i.e.*, "Yellow Fever."

The absence in Yellow Fever of any eruption, of any absolutely pathognomonic sign or symptom, and of any bacteriological test, or "reaction," renders the clinical problem very difficult, and greatly enhances the importance of the opinion of the medical attendant, assuming that he is competent, as to the nature of the disease from which the patient suffered.

When therefore cases, of one of which it is stated, "Although all the symptoms were mild it was undoubtedly a case of Yellow Fever, and the patient recovered," and of another, "he died undoubtedly of Yellow Fever," are classed as "Possible Yellow Fever, no sufficient evidence," the limitations of any conclusions as to the prevalence of the disease based upon this classification are at once obvious.

SIERRA LEONE.

1900–1909.

No case of Yellow Fever is recorded as having occurred at Sierra Leone between the years 1900 and 1909, but it is possible (*vide* Second Report, p. 108) that the death of a Syrian in 1908 and of a European in 1909 may have been really due to that disease.

1910.

The epidemic which occurred at Freetown in this year is analysed in the Second Report of the Commission (pp. 110-115), and the quarters of the town in which the patients lived are shown in the map appended to that Report. Although from lack of sufficient evidence or from the absence of a post-mortem examination, seven of the 21 cases constituting the epidemic were not classified by the Commission as Yellow Fever, there can, we think, be little doubt as to their real nature. In only two cases not included amongst the foregoing, was the local diagnosis thought to have been erroneous, and the duration of the epidemic is not affected thereby, as it was closed by two fatal cases.

1911–12–13.

There is no record of the occurrence of Yellow Fever in Sierra Leone in the years 1911–12–13.

SENEGAMBIA, SENEGAL.

1900–1913.

In the following table the incidence of the disease in Senegambia so far as it is known during the period under review is shown. It has not been thought necessary to give the localities as they are mentioned in the Second Report:—

Year.	Cases.	Deaths.
1900	416	225
1901	10	5
1902	—	—
1903	—	—
1904	Dakar declar	ed infected.
1905	2	1 ?
1906	?	21
1907	—	—
1908	—	—
1909	—	—
1910	7 ?	7 ?
1911	Dakar and Ru	fisque infected.
1912	33	25
1913	—	—

Gambia.

1900–1913.

1900.

The epidemic which occurred in the Gambia in this year is described in the Second Report (pages 57–60).

1901.

A very suspicious case of "Bilious Remittent Fever" in a Commissioner, who was travelling at the time, ended fatally.

A death from "Pernicious Malarial Fever" took place in port; the disease was contracted outside the Colony.

1902–1910.

In 1903 a member of a French Catholic Mission recently arrived from Senegal, died from a severe attack of "Bilious Remittent Fever."

In 1905 a death occurred in hospital from Malignant Fever with Hyperpyrexia.

In 1906 in a case of Malignant Remittent Fever with Hyperpyrexia it is recorded that "intra-muscular injections of quinine produced an immediate beneficial effect upon the course of the fever, causing an uninterrupted convalescence to set in."

Assuming the statement to be accurate it is clear that the case was not one of Yellow Fever.*

In the years included, but not mentioned, there is no evidence of the presence of Yellow Fever, but it is recorded under 1909 that the 151 Europeans all used mosquito nets at night, or lived in mosquito protected houses. Four Europeans, however; died as the result of malarial infection.

1911.

The epidemic at Bathurst in this year is recorded and analysed on pp. 121–124 of the Second Report, and a map is appended showing the position of the houses in which the cases occurred.

Of the 15 cases constituting the epidemic and locally diagnosed as Yellow Fever, the Commission, following the strict rules as to classification which they have imposed upon themselves, confirmed this opinion in six cases, all of which were fatal. Five cases, of which three recovered and two died, were classed as "Probably Yellow Fever," and three cases, of which one recovered and two died, as "Possibly Yellow Fever." One fatal case was classified as "negative," as there was no sufficient record and no post-mortem examination was made.

On reference to the Second Report it will be seen (p. 124) that cases 50, 51, 52, 53, and 54 "were friends and often together in the engineers' quarters" (where the outbreak commenced). The following table shows the results of the classification of these cases.

Case No.	Classification.	Result.
50	Yellow Fever	Died.
51	Yellow Fever	Died.
52	Probable Yellow Fever	Recovered.
53	Negative	Died.
54	Probable Yellow Fever	Recovered.

In dealing with cases of Yellow Fever it is obviously easier to be certain as to the fatal cases, and more particularly those in which a post-mortem examination is made, than as to those which recover, and the reason for classifying No. 53 as "Negative" was that no record

*The observations of Dr. Cachin Itriago, referred to on p. 31, have a bearing upon this point.

was available, and no post-mortem examination was made. On epidemiological grounds, however, it is as nearly certain as possible that all these patients suffered from one and the same disease.

Of case 57 it is stated that he died with "Most marked symptoms"; classification, "Probable Yellow Fever, evidence insufficient"; but he was nursed by "case 60," with whom he lived, and at a later date "case 60" was found concealed, but screened. He was to have been put on board a steamer and smuggled away, but was removed to Hospital, where he died. Classification, "Probable Yellow Fever, details insufficient."

Case 58, a Syrian, who recovered, is similarly classified and for the same reason, but he lived in the same house as case 61, who died of "Yellow Fever."

In none of the cases which occurred in this epidemic is it probable that the local diagnosis was other than correct.

Anyone who is disposed to analyse the record of the Freetown epidemic of 1910, and of the other epidemics included in this period, from the same point of view, will have no difficulty in pointing to similar results, and lest it should be attempted to use the classification as a basis for criticism of the opinions formed by the medical officers in actual contact with the cases it is desirable, in justice to them, that this should be made clear.

This single example should, therefore, suffice to relieve us from the necessity of a further detailed examination of the records of the epidemics which are dealt with in the Second Report.

1912–1913.

There is no record of any case of Yellow Fever occurring in the Gambia in these years.

Portuguese Guinea.

1900–1913.

No information, other than that given on page 64 of the Second Report, is available as to the presence of Yellow Fever in this Colony during the years under review.

In discussing the possible sites of "endemic areas" and "endemic foci" (*vide* p. 241) a reference will be found to Portuguese Guinea.

French Guinea.

1900–1913.

No further information is available.

Soudan.

1900–1913.

The possibility of an endemic area existing in the French Soudan is considered on pp. 65-67 of the Second Report of the Commission.

Liberia.

No further information has been received.

Ivory Coast.

1900–1913.

It will be noticed in reference to this Dependency* that the outbreaks have been frequent during recent years, and it is more than probable that if the whole of the facts were known it would be clear that in the intervals the absence of the disease was more apparent than real.

Gold Coast.

1900–1913.

From 1901 to 1913 there is a continuous record of the presence of Yellow Fever in the Gold Coast Colony, although (*vide* Second Report, page 75) not at one and the same place in each year.

In the analysis of the sporadic cases which have occurred since the appointment of the Commission reference will be found to the occurrence of two cases in nursing sisters at Accra in June, 1913 (*vide p.* 66).

Togoland.

1900–1913.

An impartial review of the history of this Dependency as regards Yellow Fever can lead to no other conclusion than that the disease has been present there continuously during the whole of this period, and that the German Government of the Dependency has certainly in one case deliberately concealed its existence in order to escape the necessity of quarantine (*vide* p. 68).

---

* *Vide* Second Report of Commission, p. 68.

Togoland has been without doubt an endemic area in the past and a source of danger to the neighbouring Dependencies.

It is to be hoped that its future history will present a cleaner record.

DAHOMEY.

It is known that Yellow Fever was present in this Dependency in 1905 (Second Report, p. 79), but there is no evidence of a later date available.

NIGERIA.

1900–1913.

From the Historical Retrospect contained in the Second Report it is clear that at various periods, and especially from 1860 to 1864 Yellow Fever prevailed extensively upon the coast of what is now the Southern Provinces of Nigeria (*vide* p. 85 *et seq.*). The places specially affected were Benin, Bonny, Calabar, Lagos and "all the rivers in the Bights," but from that date onwards we have no record of the continued presence of the disease in those regions.

It is interesting to note that during the epidemics of 1910, 1911 and 1912 Southern Nigeria escaped, and when the Commission were called upon to select the places to which their special Investigators should be sent, it was decided (*vide* First Report, p. 3) that: "13. As no cases of Yellow Fever had been reported from Southern Nigeria during those years, and as the Principal Medical Officer reported that no suspicious cases of fever had since occurred, no Investigators should be sent there;" yet the Commission had hardly set to work when an unexpected epidemic at Lagos rendered that place the most important field for their operations. This epidemic is described and analysed in the "Report on certain outbreaks of Yellow Fever in Lagos, 1913, and January and February, 1914," by Dr. T. M. Russell Leonard, contained in Volume I. of the Investigators' Reports, pages 207–316. Reference to this Report shows that the disease was not really absent from Southern Nigeria during the year 1910, but the true nature of two cases which occurred in natives was not realised at the time. "At Lagos, in Nigeria, there were two suspicious and rapidly fatal cases in natives. These were not reported as Yellow Fever, but from the clinical and post-mortem appearances were very probably cases of true Yellow Fever" (*vide* I.R., Vol. I., page 207). Accompanying Dr. Leonard's report is a plan of the town of Lagos, showing in *yellow* the areas which were "declared," and in which quarantine was imposed, in *blue* the areas which were considered to be suspicious, and in *red* the European quarters. Where the letter S in *green* occurs on that map it indicates the presence there of *Stegomyia* mosquitoes and larvæ.

The Lagos Epidemic of 1913 *and* 1914.

The first outbreak occurred on May 12th and lasted until the 28th, 1913, and consisted of six cases of which one, in a European, was fatal. Four mild cases occurred in natives and one of a similar character in a European, the subject of Malaria.

The second outbreak occupied the period from 16th July to 1st September. Seventeen cases occurred, of which six were in Europeans and the remainder in natives. Of the Europeans two died, of the eleven natives all recovered.

The third outbreak began on September 19th and continued up to December 25th. There were four cases in natives, all of which recovered; and eight cases in Europeans of which four proved fatal.

This gives the following totals:—

	Died.	Recovered.	Totals.
Europeans	7	8	15
Natives	—	20	20

Note.—It should be stated, however, that the Commission were not unanimous in accepting the local diagnosis of Yellow Fever in a certain proportion of these cases.

French Gaboon.

1909.

The Commission have received information shewing that Yellow Fever was prevailing at Phillipville in July, 1909.

SECTION VII.

FROM JANUARY, 1913, TO DECEMBER, 1915.

In this section we shall first give a brief account of the sporadic cases which have occurred since the appointment of the Commission.

They present many points of great interest, which repay careful study, and they indicate clearly that the disease is widely distributed in almost every Dependency.

Each sporadic case is a potential epidemic, and that they should have been so numerous whilst the epidemics have been so few, is really a tribute to the success which has attended the measures taken in each case to limit the spread of the disease.

(*A*)—ANALYSIS OF SPORADIC CASES.

(1) NIGERIA—SOUTHERN PROVINCES.

1913.

(*a*) ABEOKUTA.

Abeokuta, the capital of Egbaland, lies 7° 10′ N., 3° 23′ E., and is situated to the north of Lagos town and island. It is enclosed by the districts of Ibadan, Ikorodu, Lagos, Badagri and Meko. The area is approximately 3,420 acres, and the population is about 51,255. The town is 62 miles by railway from Lagos, and 65½ miles from Ibadan. Badagri is 72 miles, and Ikorodu 50 miles distant by road.

The case of Mr. Brooks, of Abeokuta, was one of the first to be investigated by the Commission, and on account of its importance a special enquiry was ordered, and was efficiently carried out by Dr. E. J. Wyler, whose report will be found in Volume I. of the Investigators' Reports (page 3). As the facts of the case are given in detail in Dr. Leonard's Report (Investigators' Reports, Vol. I., page 216), it will be sufficient to state here that the patient, a European trader, aged 28, had been continuously resident in Abeokuta for three months prior to his death, with the single exception of a visit to

Lagos in February, 1913. He was taken ill on Saturday, May 10th, 1913, on the evening of his arrival at Lagos, where he had gone for a change, having been out of sorts for three days previously. He was admitted to the Lagos Hospital on May 12th, and died there from Yellow Fever on May 14th. It is clear that this patient must have been infected in Abeokuta, but the disease was not known to be present there, and the investigation did not reveal the occurrence of suspicious cases of fever amongst the natives shortly before the patient's illness.

The number of Europeans resident in Abeokuta in May, 1913, was 32. No suspicious cases of illness had occurred amongst them during the preceding twelve months. Six of them may possibly have been immune to Yellow Fever, as they had previously resided in regions where Yellow Fever is endemic, before coming to West Africa, although, as none of them had suffered from that disease, it is not very likely that they were insusceptible; the others had been in West Africa for periods varying from 40 months to two months.

Abeokuta forms part of the Egba native state, and the sanitary conditions in the town are apparently very defective. *Stegomyia* larvæ were found in most of the water tanks examined. This patient's house was surrounded by native compounds. The European community, although small in numbers, was quite sufficiently large to have afforded evidence of the presence of an active endemic focus of Yellow Fever had such existed for any lengthened period, more especially as there was no European reservation. The only evidence of the possible existence of such a focus is furnished by the fact that in February, 1912, and in July, 1912, two Europeans, recently arrived at Lagos from Abeokuta, were admitted to Hospital suffering from illness diagnosed as Malaria, but presenting features of a suspicious character (*vide* I.R., Vol. I., page 13, table 3, Dr. Wyler's Report No. 1). In both these cases albuminuria was present. In the first the pulse on admission to hospital was 50, there was marked tenderness in the epigastrium, the liver and spleen were palpable; there is no record of the condition of the blood. In the second, the pulse on admission was 72, the spleen was palpable, Widal negative; the temperature was not reduced by quinine; no parasites were found in the blood. Recovery followed in each case after an illness in hospital lasting 13 days.

The virus may have been introduced into Abeokuta from Lagos, distant 64 miles, and reached by rail in a journey of from three to four hours. The average number of natives travelling daily between Abeokuta and Iddo (the railway terminus for Lagos) during March, April and May, 1913, was found to be 110. It is stated that such passengers usually carry with them as much baggage as the regulations permit.

That Lagos was a possible source from which infection was carried to Abeokuta follows from the fact that, shortly after this patient's death, cases of Yellow Fever began to be noted amongst natives in Lagos (*vide* cases 2, 3 and 4, I.R., Vol. 1, page 223). One of these patients (case 2) was taken ill on May 7th; a second on May 9th, and a third on May 10th. In each case recovery followed after an illness lasting from 15 to 17 days. Such cases may have been occurring previously, as until the death of Mr. Brooks, attention had not been drawn to the presence of Yellow Fever. Lagos must therefore be regarded as having been in May, 1913, an endemic area, and capable of acting as the source from which infection could be conveyed to Abeokuta. Dr. Wyler investigated the possibility of the disease having been introduced into Abeokuta viâ the Dahomey-Nigeria boundary. There is constant traffic between Dahomey and Abeokuta, and at all the important towns, where traders would be most likely to stop, *Stegomyia* were found in abundance, but his enquiries did not elicit any facts of importance. Whether the disease was endemic in Abeokuta or was introduced shortly before the occurrence of Mr. Brooks' illness cannot be decided, but it is evident that it did not die out immediately, as Dr. Wyler was informed by the Father Superior of the French Catholic Mission at Abeokuta some weeks subsequently to his visit, that another undoubted case of Yellow Fever had occurred there, the patient being a Syrian.

This case is described in Dr. Wyler's Third Report (I.R., Vol. I., page 36), from which it appears that:—

(1) The illness began on July 31st. On the seventh day there was a measles-like rash over the face and body, petechial in places.

(2) The patient had not been away from Abeokuta for many months, except to visit Lagos about the end of April, and Ibadan about the middle of June.

(3) No suspicious cases had occurred at Abeokuta since that of Mr. Brooks.

(4) The patient had not been inside a native house for at least two years.

(5) He lived alone and had no servant.

(6) Two months before his illness another Syrian trader came to stay with him and remained for three months, being in good health all the time. This man's luggage consisted of a small handbag containing clothes.

(7) The patient's house was in a thickly populated part of the town, surrounded by native compounds.

It would appear that in this case, as in that of Mr. Brooks, the infection must have come from a native source.

It is possible that the illness from which the three natives suffered whose cases are described in Dr. Wyler's Third Report (I.R., Vol. I., page 39) was Yellow Fever, but the details given are insufficient to support a definite diagnosis, and the cases were not observed by a medical man. They occurred on July 1st, August 6th, and August 10th, all were cases of fever attended with albuminuria, which disappeared at the end of the illness.

(*b*) OGBOMOSHO.

Ogbomosho, a town in the Oshogbo Sub-District of the Southern Provinces of Nigeria from which it is distant some 43 miles, lies 8° 8′ N., 4° 15′ E. It is 62 miles from Ibadan, and has a population of 80,000.

On August 22nd, 1913, a patient was admitted to Lagos Hospital L. 54.
whose case formed the subject of a special inquiry by Dr. E. J. Wyler (I.R., Vol. 1, p. 30, Report No. 2).

At that period all passengers arriving at Lagos by train were subjected to medical examination with a view to the detection of cases of fever, especially Yellow Fever. The patient, a male native, aged 20, was found to have a temperature of 103° F., and was therefore detained. He suffered from an illness which, in the opinion of the majority of the Commission, was an attack of mild Yellow Fever ending in recovery.

This patient had come to Lagos from Ogbomosho, which is described as a large and dirty town of about 80,000 inhabitants, situated on an extensive lofty plateau about 180 miles from Lagos and 30 miles from the nearest railway station.

He had been in Ogbomosho for one month prior to setting out for Lagos, to which place he travelled viâ Oyo, Fiditi and Ibadan (three days). He remained there overnight and left on the following day by train for Lagos (about seven hours' journey).

Dr. Wyler's enquiries at Ogbomosho, Oyo, Fiditi and Ibadan failed to elicit any evidence of the existence of present or past suspicious cases of fever, or of a suspicious high mortality among native adults or children. An American Baptist Medical Missionary who had resided at Ogbomosho continuously for two and a half years, and carried on a dispensary there, had not met with any cases of the kind. No suspicious cases amongst Europeans had occurred at either Ogbomosho or Oyo. At the former place there were three European non-officials, and at Oyo twelve. All the Europeans at Ogbomosho live in one household.

The patient on admission to hospital was considered from his symptoms to be in the third or fourth day of the disease (5th day, Dr. Wyler's Report, p. 33). In that case he must have been infected at Ogbomosho.

Commentary.

This case is of great importance both in its epidemiological and clinical aspects.

The following points are worthy of notice:—

(1) The patient was a native, and had been resident for one month in a large native town, which was not known to harbour the disease.

(2) No suspicious cases amongst either the natives or Europeans had been observed in that place or in any other town visited by the patient.

(3) He was, although a native, not immune to the disease, but the attack was not of a severe type, and the illness ended in recovery.

(4) He was sufficiently well to be travelling on business, and on admission to hospital did not complain of more urgent symptoms than headache and pains in the limbs.

(5) The patient was the subject of malarial infection, as so often occurs in native cases.

(6) Lastly, it is almost certain that had it not been for the quarantine examination at Ebute-Metta the case would have escaped recognition.

(c) LAGOS.

The following is classified by the Commission as a case of "Possible Yellow Fever." It is given in detail in Dr. Wyler's Report No. 1, Appendix 3 (*vide* Vol. I., I.R., p. 27), and is mentioned there as of "special interest" as illustrating the difficulty attending medical investigation among the natives in the "bush."

"APPENDIX III.

"The patient was a woman aet. about 20 years, the illness had began with frontal headache and vomiting after food. When first seen she had been ill six days; there was no headache, but she felt, and looked, very ill.

"Temperature normal.

"Pulse 80.

"No jaundice.

"Tongue clean.

"Spleen not enlarged.

"Bowels open normally.

"No frequency of micturition.

"No œdema.

"Heart and lungs normal.

"Urine: Thick cloud of albumen and bile present.

"*On the following day.*

"Slight yellowish tinge of conjunctiva.

"Urine: Albumen less in amount: no bile.

"General condition better. No pyrexia.

"*Next day.*

"Conjunctival tinge of jaundice as before.

"Urine: Albumen lessening.

"General condition much improved.

"*Commentary.*

"The record of this case investigated in the 'bush' is necessarily incomplete. I have no doubt that it was not a case of renal disease or of malaria, and I quote it because it appears to come into line with the cases mentioned in my Commentary in Appendix I."

(*d*) CALABAR.

In the following case the Commission were unable to arrive at a positive diagnosis of Yellow Fever, from defects in the evidence.

It is classified as "Probable Yellow Fever."

The patient, a Russian Finn, aet. 21, a fireman on board the ss. "Monrovia," was admitted 26th October, 1913, to the Calabar Hospital. He was unable to speak either English, German or French, and no interpreter was available. The illness commenced suddenly on Sunday, 26th October, 1913, with fever (T. over 105° F.), and severe bilious vomiting. On admission face flushed; eyes injected; frontal and occipital headache; pulse 80, low tension; epigastric tenderness. Liver not enlarged; spleen slightly so. No albuminuria; no malaria parasites.

"*27th October.*—Faget's sign noted: no vomiting, no albuminuria: bile pigment in urine.

"*28th October.*—Albumen slight: quantity of urine diminished: jaundice slight.

"*29th October.*—No albumen: jaundice persists.

"*30th October.*—Albumen again present: whitish bile-stained fluid vomited.

"*31st October.*—Albumen disappeared: jaundice still present. Four observations of the pulse varied from 62 to 64.

"Convalescent."

The local diagnosis was "Yellow Fever."

(*e*) WARRI.

1913.

An outbreak of Yellow Fever which occurred at Warri in May and June, 1913, was investigated by Dr. E. J. Wyler, and forms the subject of Section I. of his 4th Report (I.R., Vol. 1, p. 44).

Commentary.

The points of interest in connection with this outbreak are as follows:—

(1) Both the patients were Europeans engaged at a store, living in the same house in the compound of the firm in whose employment they were.

(2) The first case, which terminated fatally, occurred on 22nd May, 1913. The second, which ended in recovery, occurred on June 10th.

(3) No evidence was obtained after a most exhaustive inquiry of the occurrence of any cases of Yellow Fever, or even of suspicious cases of fever, in the town of Warri, or the district in which it is situated, or amongst the Europeans (4), or native employees (40) of the firm, and no exceptional mortality had occurred in the district.

(4) The first case (L.26) had not been away from Warri for three months prior to his illness; the second case (L.34) had not been away for one month.

(5) Case L.26 had always used a mosquito net, but on the night of May 26th—five days before he became ill—he slept on the verandah without a net, and was so much bitten by mosquitoes that in the morning his face and arms were swollen. Case L.34 always slept under a mosquito net, but occasionally arose at daybreak and lay outside the net upon a sofa.

(6) Case L.26 (fatal) was in his first tour, and had been on the coast for eighteen months. The patient who recovered (L.34) had been some years in West Africa, and was in the sixth month of his tour.

(7) After the removal to hospital of Case L.26, the second patient (L.34) worked in the evening in the store—which was infested with mosquitoes—in which the first patient had previously worked, and as he was taken ill twenty days later, it is probable that he was infected by mosquitoes which had bitten the first patient.

(8) No cases of Yellow Fever or of any disease resembling it occurred at Warri subsequent to those here described.

Conclusion.

The conclusion to be drawn from the occurrence of these cases is that Warri was at that time an endemic focus of Yellow Fever, and that no definite evidence of the fact was manifest until a European became infected.

Dr. Wyler investigated the clinical and post-mortem records at Warri from January, 1911, to October, 1913, with a view to ascertain if any mild or typical cases of Yellow Fever had been mistaken for cases of Malaria. Two cases which occurred on March 6th and 7th, 1912, are described in the Report, and the temperature charts are given. In each of these cases albuminuria was present, and it is stated that "the pulse-rate was suggestive," but no record of the pulse appears in either case.

The Report contains a valuable analysis of the cases of Malaria accompanied by albuminuria, a subject which is considered at length at a later stage of this Report (*vide* p. 168).

ONITSHA.

The following case was classified by the Commission as "Possible Yellow Fever."

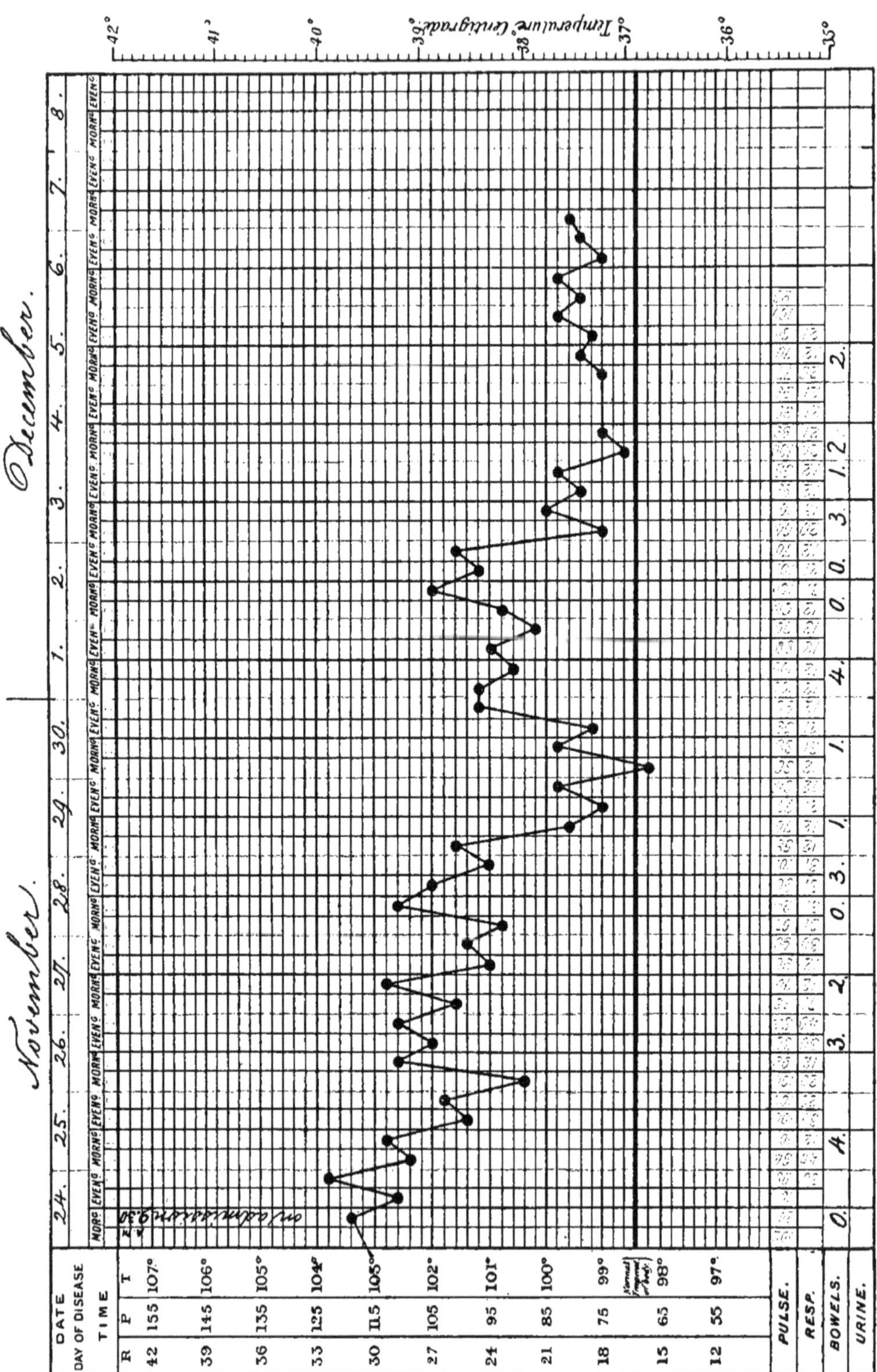

"ONITSHA—CENTRAL PROVINCE.

"7th December, 1913.

"*Report on a suspicious case of Yellow Fever.*

"On the 24th November, 1913, a case was admitted into the Native hospital, and believed by me to be an ordinary case of Malarial Fever, and for two days was treated as such, when the cause of the disease began to diverge widely in point of character from Malaria, and eventually turned out to be what, in my opinion, was Yellow Fever.

"Male native, apparent age 25 years, a native of Itbobo behind Asaba, a man who had recently been appointed as gang-driver to the Onitsha Prisons.

"Admitted to hospital 24th November, 1913. T. 103·4° F., P. 102. Headache and bodily pains. He was given 10 grains of quinine immediately, phenacetin, caffein, and an aperient, and nursed as usual.

"It was not until the evening of the 26th that my attention was particularly called to his case when, in spite of 15 grains of quinine a day having been taken, and other treatment, his temperature remained up, but apart from physical signs his bodily distress was greatly accentuated. T. 102·6° F., P. 6, Resp. 40. Tongue covered with thin whitish-grey fur, but clean all round the edges, and markedly tremulous; his limbs were tremulous, his skin was dry, hot and pungent. On examination of the urine, I found well-marked albuminuria. The eyes were normal in colour. The liver was apparently normal; the bowels had reacted to an aperient, but were otherwise constipated. I injected intra-muscularly 10 grains of quinine, but just as quinine had failed to improve matters before, this also failed. His chest was normal on stethoscopic examination. He dozed or slept a good deal, and was always a little delirious in his sleep. The fever was of the asthenic type when quite awake, and he preferred sitting up in bed, was very restless, and constantly the limbs shook.

"The chart, which was faithfully kept throughout, shows no morning or evening rise or fall, neither do I think the temperature or symptoms were very much affected at any time by the exhibition of quinine or any other drug. It is certainly the first case of its kind I have ever seen, and on instigating a thorough enquiry, I elicited the following facts:—

"The patient says that:—

"He has never had the disease (himself) before but he knows it quite well, and after repeated sifting of the evidence he was emphatic about its differing entirely from ordinary Malarial Fever, and that it is never associated with any bowel or lung, or ordinary well-known complaint of everyday occurrence.

"The cases in his district, Asaba, had occurred about every three years, and about six or eight people only had suffered at the time.

"The native doctors know a remedy which I tried to find out, but failed to do so.

"To-day, December 7th, 1913, albuminuria is still present, but not so well marked as yesterday, and to-day I applied Gmelin's test for the bile pigments.

"The test gave a much blacker reaction in the presence of the HNO_3 than is usually obtained, *i.e.*, a darkish purple, and I am not convinced therefore of the reliability of my experiment. The patient is rapidly approaching convalescence, and for several days his appetite has been very good.

"I should like an expression of opinion on this case.

"Every prisoner has been under observation since, every man being personally examined, and every possible precaution has been taken to avoid infection. No other case has come under my notice since.

"M.O., Onitsha.

"7th December, 1913.

"P.S.—Other points of interest suggested by the Provincial Medical Officer and replied to herein:—

"*Frontal Headache.*—Yes, this was present in a most marked degree.

"*Epigastric Distress.*—Was not marked, but the patient lay for some days coiled up during the asthenic stage in a manner suggestive of abdominal pain.

"*Vomiting.*—Yes, vomiting was present, not coffee-ground, but of a darkish green tint.

"*Conjunctivæ.*—No ferret-eyed appearance obtained, but a jaundiced appearance supervened as the disease neared its termination.

"*Deafness.*—I did not ask.

"*Pulse rate.*—The chart speaks for itself.

"*Malarial Fever.*—The question was not eliminated by the microscope. Quinine in large doses and hypodermically did not influence the temperature or disease.

"*Albuminuria* has now ceased.

"The patient is now convalescent and about to be discharged.

"Medical Officer, Onitsha."

(II) GOLD COAST.

(*a*) ACCRA.

1913.

Accra, the headquarters of the Gold Coast Government, is situated on the coast, and lies 5° 32′ N., 0° 57′ W.

On reference to the Second Report of the Commission (p. 119) it will be seen that an outbreak of Yellow Fever occurred at Accra in 1911. There is no record of the reappearance of the disease there in 1912.

CHRISTIANSBORG, ACCRA.

1913.

Two "Probable" cases of Yellow Fever occurred in Government House, Christiansborg, in March, 1913. Both ended in recovery. The first was of a moderately severe type; the second of a mild type. They do not call for any special comment. Both patients were "new-comers," having arrived in the Colony on December 26th, 1912.

Five cases of a mild type subsequently occurred at Accra in the same month in natives; all ended in recovery.

ACCRA.

March, 1913.

The following case in a native boy which occurred at Accra was classified by the Commission as "Probably Yellow Fever."

Case 3.—March 31st, 1913. Quey, male, aet. 5, native of Accra, was seen by a local native practitioner in a comatose state after a few hours' illness, dying shortly after. A post-mortem was held, which showed signs highly suspicious of Yellow Fever, but failing a history and previous symptoms it was not accepted as such, although the premises were fumigated, and the other residents kept under observation for six days. No other cases of pyrexia occurred here. Diagnosis, probably Yellow Fever.

> "Patient's name, Quey. Age, five years. Male. Ill five days. Onset with chill, afterwards skin very hot. Slight vomiting, but no description of vomited matter. Great restlessness. Did not stay in bed. Bowels constipated. Did not take food.
>
> "Very slight greenish yellow tint of sclerotics.
>
> "Post-mortem rigidity absent.
>
> "Congestion of tissues on section.
>
> "*Lungs* congested, but no areas of consolidation. Patechiæ on pleuræ.
>
> "*Heart*, white clot in ventricle (left). Patechiæ on pericardium.
>
> "*Liver* congested and yellowish brown.
>
> "*Spleen* not markedly enlarged. 'Sago' appearance on section.
>
> "*Kidneys* very intensely congested. Capsule stripped easily.

" *Stomach.*—Submucous hæmorrhages on greater curvature at pyloric end. Stomach empty.

" *Intestines.*—Submucous hæmorrhages in first part of duodenum, rest of intestine normal in appearance. Intestinal contents not red or black (greyish yellow). Two *Ascaris lumbricoides.*

" *Brain* congested.

" *Bladder* empty.

" *Smears.*—*Brain* smear (pia arachnoid): No parasites, no pigment.

" *Liver* smear: Hepatic cells intensely fatty. Connective tissue cells with pigment. No parasites.

" *Spleen* smear: No parasites, slight amount of pigment. No plague bacilli.

" I consider that Yellow Fever was the cause of death."

Two cases of Yellow Fever occurred in June, 1913; both the patients were nursing sisters, residing in the Wesleyan Girls' School. One case terminated fatally, the other in recovery, after a severe illness. The patient who died had only arrived from England 14 days before the onset of her illness; the other was in her second tour of service, of which she had completed 10 months.

(*b*) CAPE COAST.

1913.

This case was classified by the Commission as "Possible Yellow Fever."

One reason for mentioning it here is to illustrate the type of case which has been included under that heading.

The patient was a native official aet. 58.

The illness was of a sudden onset with rigor, pyrexia, nausea, headache and moderate epigastric tenderness. The patient looked ill on admission to hospital, and the conjunctivæ were deep yellow. The finger nails also showed a light tinge of yellow. It will be remembered that this latter sign was present in a marked degree in the case of Dr. Lundie (*vide* p. 72). Albumen was present in the urine on the third day, and persisted until the 8th or 9th day. No malarial parasites were found, and quinine had no effect upon the temperature. On the 4th day there was vomiting "once of strings of mucus tinged with fresh blood and glistening yellow particles." Faget's sign was not present, and the pulse was quick. Typhoid was negatived by the examination of the blood.

Recovery took place after an illness lasting from June 19th to July 12th. The pulse rate was 100 on his return from a holiday after the illness.

(c) ABOKOBI.

1913.

Abokobi is a native village, situated about 13 miles from Accra; it lies 5° 42′ N., 0° 20′ W.

A fatal case of Yellow Fever in a European was reported from here in May, 1913. The patient was a German, a member of the Basel Mission. He had been in the country since January, 1913; is said never to have had fever, and to have taken quinine regularly. He was taken ill on May 10th, and died with typical symptoms on May 15th.

No further cases occurred, and the source of the infection was not discovered. The movements of the patient preceding the onset of his illness are not recorded.

The following are taken from a list of deaths of Europeans at Abokobi since 1856, which contains 22 names, of whom 7 are infants.

No.	Name.	Age.	Died.	Cause of Death.
8	John Uric Luthy ...	29	1869	Climatic Fever.
11	Fred. August Ehmer	33	1878	Gall Fever.
14	C. Berck	32	1883	Gall Fever.
15	Johannes Schmid...	25	1885	Stroke after preceding Fever.
17	Lydia V. Serger ...	31	1888	Bilious Fever.
18	Emmanuel Serger...	2	1891	Fever complicated with sunstroke.

(d) QUITTAH.

1913.

Quittah is a station on the seaboard of the Gold Coast. It lies 5° 55′ N., 1° 0′ E., and is situated on a long strip of land of two to three miles in width which separates the lagoon from the sea.

Case 1.—The patient, Quarshie Kpoha, age 19, was a native who had always been resident at Quittah, but was in Lome, Togoland, for two days. The illness began on May 9th, two days after his return home. He lived in a part of the town called Alata, under the wall of the Bremen Sisters' house. Recovery followed after a mild attack, lasting eleven days. All the inhabitants were kept under observation, but no other suspicious case occurred immediately.

In June, however, the disease reappeared and proved fatal in *Case* 2, a clergyman, aet. 27, the head of the Bremen Mission School. This patient visited Anyako on June 21st, and remained there until June 23rd, when he returned to Quittah. The illness commenced on June 29th, and death took place on the evening of the fourth day.

A careful investigation of the circumstances was made, but the direct connection between this case and the preceding was not made out.

It is stated in the report that "in the compound in which the case of the missionary occurred 29 natives resided and 294 boys attended school daily." The compound itself lies in the midst of a congested native quarter.

Twenty-nine adult Europeans were resident in Quittah in June, 1913.

The following further extracts from this report are worthy of record:—

"The Government of Togoland (German) placed Quittah and the ports of Denu and Addah in quarantine, and established a cordon on the frontier, beyond which no one was allowed to pass until he or she had been kept under surveillance for five days, in buildings erected for the purpose."

"It seems hard that this Colony should be thus penalised for being honest enough to declare a case of Yellow Fever, when there is no reason to suppose that the disease is any less endemic across the border than it is here, and in this connection I invite attention to the attached description by Dr. Le Fanu (Appendix V.) of a case of Yellow Fever which occurred in Lome in May last, and was not reported to this Government."

"APPENDIX V.

"SENIOR SANITARY OFFICER,

"Mr. Mahuken, an agent for A. Kulenkamp, in Keta, gave me the following history of his illness in May, 1913:—

"Left Anecho May 14th; he arrived Lome same day. Left Lome Thursday, May 15th, and arrived Atakpanu same day. Taken ill Monday, 19th May; very ill Tuesday; proceeded to Lome on Wednesday; seen by Dr. Kruger on Thursday, 22nd, who immediately had him removed to hospital; *locked Mr. Mahuken's room, and said no one was to enter it until it had been fumigated.*"

"*Illness*: 19*th May*.—Headache and fever. Headache described as 'strong rush of blood to the head.'

"*20th*.—Feeling very ill. Headache, fever, and rigors.

"*21st*.—To Lome. Condition no better. Jaundice and vomiting.

"*22nd*.—To hospital. Marked jaundice. Vomit getting very dark until it was described by Dr. Kruger as bluish-black-brown. Urine contained cylinders (casts). The pulse became very slow, at one time sinking to 32. At the onset of the illness there was much diarrhœa, which ceased as the vomiting became copious.

"Patient, while in hospital, was isolated in a mosquito-proof room. He was not then, or later, informed of the nature of his illness, but is certain it was Yellow Fever.

"I think there is little doubt that his surmise is correct.

"G. E. H. LE FANU.

"*22nd July*, 1913."

It will be seen that Quarshie Kpoba was in Lome on May 7th. Mr. Mahuken was probably infected either at Anecho or at Lome, at both of which places he was on May 14th. There was therefore a focus of Yellow Fever at one or both of those places at that date.

This case, the existence of which would not otherwise have been revealed, is of great importance and almost certainly proves that the native Quarshie Kpoba was infected in Lome, and that the Government of Togoland were concealing the existence of the disease.

In a memorandum by the Senior Sanitary Officer dated May 21st, 1913, the case of Quarshie Kpoba is thus referred to:—

> "It will be interesting to see the report. This looks like a case of *Atridi asara*. variously translated by the natives as bilious fever and yellow fever—probably true yellow fever. There are a number of records of death from it in the cemetery register at Abokobi, to which I have called the attention of the Investigators."

The Cemetery Register of Abokobi.

A copy of this Register has been obtained, and proves to be a document of some interest. The Commission are indebted to Mr. H. S. Newlands, Private Secretary to the Governor of the Gold Coast, for undertaking the translation of it from the German, in which a large number of the entries were made. In cases in which the native names of the diseases were used, these have been translated by the Chief Dispenser, an educated native. In the copy furnished to the Commission the entry "Atridi" occurs eight times in the years 1882, 1883, and 1884, and it is only during those years that the entries are given in the native language (Ga). The entry "Atridi asara" does not appear in the copy, but when these words occur in the original it seems that they have been translated "Bilious Fever," as we are informed that "Yellow Fever" is a translation of an entry "Gelbfieber." Also, that when the word "Atridi" stands alone it should be translated "Malaria," and in the years just mentioned the eight entries appear in the copy thus: "Atridi (Malaria)," but that "Atridi asara" may be translated either "Yellow Fever" or "Bilious Fever." It is suggested that entries were made in the German, and also in the native language, because the Register was kept at the Basel Mission, and some of the missionaries may not have known the European equivalent for the native names, or possibly, the Register may have been from time to time in charge of a native. It appears to be doubtful whether the entries were made by a medical man.

The Register covers a period of 50 years, *i.e.*, from 1865 to 1914, and contains 338 entries.

In the year 1874 sixteen deaths were registered, the largest number in any one year; none of these, however, were due to "Yellow Fever." That disease appears to have been present in the following years, viz., 1893, 1894, 1895, 1896 and 1913, in each of which a single death is recorded from it.

The following are given as examples of the entries. The names and parentage have been omitted:—

1886.

	Age.	*Date.*	*Cause of death.*
1.	About 5 years ...	May 27 ...	Fever.
2.	29 years, 8 months	April 17 ...	Fever preceded by childbed.
3.	About 73½ years ...	May 22 ...	Fever.
4.	Age omitted ...	Aug. 5 ...	Bilious Fever.
5.	,, ,, ...	,, 19 ...	Bilious Fever.
6.	About 46 years ...	Sept. 19 ...	(Cause omitted.)
7.	15 years, 10 months	Nov. 17 ...	Sunstroke.

1888.

	Age.	*Date.*	*Cause of death.*
1.	31 years	Jan. 6 ...	Bilious Fever.
2.	6 years, 10 months	April 22 ...	Bilious Fever.
3.	2 years, 18 days ...	July 12 ...	Bilious Fever.
4.	7 months, 2 days...	Nov. 7 ...	Bilious Fever.
5.	56 years, 5 months	,, 12 ...	Rheumatic Fever.
6.	Age omitted ...	July (?) ...	Madness.

1893.

	Age.		*Date.*		*Cause of death.*
1.	Age omitted	...	Feb. 18	...	Fever.
2.	About 65 years	...	June 19	...	Strong Fever and Dropsy.
3.	" 48 "	...	" 24	...	Yellow Fever.
4.	" 13 "	...	July 24	...	Fever complicated with cramp or sunstroke.
5.	" 57 "	...	" 27	...	Fever.
6.	" 3 "	...	" 28	...	Fever.
7.	" 63 "	...	Sept. 28	...	Bilious Fever.
8.	" 4 "	...	" 29	...	Fever.
9.	" 4 "	...	Oct. 12	...	Fever and Dysentery.
10.	" 25 "	...	Nov. 16	...	Belly-ache.
11.	" 28 "	...	" 30	...	Bilious Fever.
12.	" 3½ "	...	Dec. 10	...	Dysentery.

The following table gives the total number of entries of certain febrile diseases:—

Climatic Fever	1
Yellow Fever	5
Fever	30
Bilious Fever	29
Atridi (Malaria)	8
Dysentery	27

Such entries as "Strong Diarrhœa" and "Bowels complaint" are of frequent occurrence.

It is a curious fact that 13 deaths are attributed to Sunstroke.

The incidence of Tuberculosis does not come within the scope of this enquiry, but as the possible increase of that disease of late amongst the natives is often under discussion it may be of interest to mention that in this Register 24 deaths are attributed to it.

We are clearly not justified in regarding this Register as containing an accurate statement of the facts as to the causes of death during the last fifty years of the persons whose names appear therein, but taking the evidence for what it may be considered to be worth it would appear:—

1. That during the years 1893, 1894, 1895, 1896, and 1913 Yellow Fever was present there, *i.e.*, 17 years prior to the outbreak at Sierra Leone in 1910, which drew attention to the fact of its existence on the Coast and led to the appointment of the Commission.

2. That diseases known as "Fever" and "Bilious Fever" were much more prevalent over the whole period of fifty years.
3. That the words "Atridi asara," in the Ga language, may be correctly translated as either "Bilious Fever" or "Yellow Fever."
4. That the word "Atridi" standing alone, signifies "Malaria" and appears much less often than "Atridi asara," signifying either "Yellow Fever" or "Bilious Fever."
5. That at least three types of acute febrile disease were recognised, but that whether they differed in kind or only in severity cannot be determined.
6. That in one and the same year "Yellow Fever," "Bilious Fever" and "Fever," are often found in association, *i.e.*: —
1893. Yellow Fever (1), Bilious Fever (2), Fever (7).
1894. Yellow Fever (1), Bilious Fever (2), Fever (4).

(*e*) BOLE.

1913.

Bole, a town in the Northern Territories of the Gold Coast, is situated some 12 miles from the Black Volta river, which in that region separates the Northern Territories from the neighbouring French possessions. It lies 90° 2′ N., 2° 25′ W.

Two, and possibly four, cases of Yellow Fever occurred there in September and October, 1913.

One member of the Commission, who was not present at the meeting at which this and the following case were classified as "Yellow Fever," subsequently on reading the reports dissented from that view.

The first patient, Dr. Lundie, West African Medical Staff, had been stationed at Bole for seven months, and had been well most of the time. He had been out for three tours. His illness commenced on September 6th, 1913, and after a prolonged attack ended in recovery on September 27th. Dr. Lundie's case was remarkable for the deep yellow pigmentation at the root of the finger nails of both hands. He showed great fortitude of mind during the illness, and for five days was assiduously attended by Mr. Sherriff, the Assistant District Commissioner, who carried out the treatment suggested by the patient.

The second case was that of Dr. R. Mugliston, West African Medical Staff, who was instructed to proceed to Bole on the receipt of the news of Dr. Lundie's illness. On September 18th he made a forced march of 70 miles to Bole to attend Dr. Lundie. He had to negotiate several swamps and rivers and was drenched by tornadoes, being wet most of the time on that march.

On October 4th he was taken ill, and suffered from a severe attack of Yellow Fever lasting 13 days; recovery was followed by a slow convalescence.

Both these patients were undoubtedly infected at Bole. Dr. Lundie stated on his return that the natives knew of the disease as a fatal one, and avoided his bungalow during his illness.

He also mentioned that there was much traffic on the road from Bole to Kintampo and on to Coomassie.

Dr. H. S. Coghill, one of the Investigators of the Commission, was sent to Bole to investigate the cases of Dr. Lundie and Dr. Mugliston.

He left Seccondee on October 12th and arrived at Kintampo on October 23rd, eight days after the death from Yellow Fever of Mr. B., a European.

He was unable to find *Stegomyia* larvæ or pupæ in nine bottles collected for his examination at Kintampo, and was informed that from a former record of mosquitoes no *Stegomyia* had ever been reported as being found in Kintampo.

The following extracts are from Dr. Coghill's report:—

"On Sunday, October 26th, I left for Bole, arriving there on Friday, the 31st, in time to see the two patients, Drs. Lundie and Mugliston, before they started for Seccondee, having been invalided by the Medical Officer in charge.

"The same day a constable brought in word to the Commissioner that fifteen natives had died at Larabanga, a village some four days' march upon one of the main roads from Bole.

"Dr. Telfer, the Medical Officer, and myself therefore left to investigate this on the following Sunday.

"Upon arriving at the village we were informed by the Chief that there had been no deaths there for some months, and no sickness for six weeks. A thorough inspection of the village was carried out by us, including a visit to the burial ground, where no evidence of any recent internment was forthcoming.

"Larvæ were collected, but no *Stegomyia* were found amongst the number.

"Meanwhile, a messenger had been sent into Bole to bring back the constable who had brought in the report.

"Upon his arrival he was interviewed, together with the Chief. As both persisted in their original statements, and having procured all the information possible, we returned to Bole, bringing in the Chief for the Commissioner to deal with.

"In Bole itself the native village is situated some 350 yards from the European quarters.

"Between these and about 200 yards from the latter are housed the constabulary and their families. No natives except personal servants are nearer the Europeans. All native compounds and houses have been visited by us in the hope of discovering any cases of sickness, which might not have been reported to the Medical Officer.

"This was all the more necessary owing to the fact that the number of patients attending the dispensary does not average two a day. Several cases of dysentery were discovered, and one of pneumonia, but all the others were of a surgical nature.

"From a record of those attending the hospital here, and from information gathered from the dispenser and others, two cases of a suspicious nature were said to have attended hospital in August and September of this year.

"Both cases were marked as suffering from fever.

"No further notes of their illness could be found, but by means of their names the cases were traced to two native policemen, who fortunately were still in Bole.

"The Commissioner kindly had them brought to the hospital, thus enabling the attached details of their illness as furnished by themselves and the dispenser to be taken down in writing.

"It seems a pity that one has to be content with details of their symptoms as gained above, but as Dr. Lundie first complained of being unwell on the 8th September, and his was an undoubted case of Yellow Fever, I think one is justified in surmising that these two cases were also due to Yellow Fever, and that in all probability the source of Dr. Lundie's infection originated from them.

"Thus Policeman Imoru Grunshi (Case No. 1), after an absence of nine days, arrived back in Bole from the Wa Road on the 24th August, and felt unwell the same evening.

"The following morning he saw the Medical Officer in charge.

"On the 5th September Policeman Ali Grunshi (Case No. 2) reported himself sick. On the 8th September Dr. Lundie went down with Yellow Fever, and on the 1st October Dr. Mugliston, who arrived in the station on the 18th September, was the last to be attacked with this disease. There has been no rain in the station now over a month, and no further cases have occurred.

"I had intended on the 24th November to visit and make an inspection of the villages in which Policeman Imoru Grunshi slept prior to his return to Bole, hoping thus to still further trace the source of the outbreak, and to furnish details of the same in this report.

"Word has, however, come to-day (22nd November) from Tumu that a European is suffering from a disease which is thought to be Yellow Fever. I am therefore setting out for that station on the 24th, and as I shall be passing through Wa I still hope to be able to inspect and make inquiries at these villages: this means that all the villages on the main roads in the Bole district will have been investigated."

"*CASE No.* 1.

"Imoru Grunshi, Policeman No. 409, native of Gyfasi, Northern Territories, Gold Coast.

"Has been in Bole five months.

"Is now in perfect health.

"History of case as obtained from patient himself on the 19th November, 1913:—

"Patient first fell ill on the 25th August, 1913, and reported himself sick the same day to the doctor.

"He first complained of frontal headache, associated with a marked rigor, following by a feeling of heat—'his skin live for hurt him.' Photophobia was also an outstanding feature.

"Epigastric pain and tenderness then became marked, and on the second day of illness vomiting set in, especially after drinking. (He was unable to take any form of solid food).

"This was at first of a bilious nature, but soon took on a very black character, lasting four days.

"His motions were normal in frequency, rather fluid and mixed with very black matter, finally becoming black altogether.

"His urine soon took on a light reddish appearance, but never black. No bleeding from gums was noticed.

"No record of jaundice, temperature, pulse, examination of blood or urine could be found.

"No further details of case could be ascertained from the patient himself.

"Patient was discharged cured on the 5th September, 1913."

"*CASE No.* 2.

"Bole, 20th November, 1913.

"Ali Grunshi, Policeman No. 306, native of Nortori, Northern Territories, Gold Coast.

"Has been in Bole 3½ months. Is now in perfect health.

" History of case as obtained from patient himself on the 18th November, 1913:—

" Patient first felt ill on the 5th September, 1913, and reported himself sick to the doctor the same day.

" He first complained of a rigor, cold, following by hot feeling all over.

" This was associated with marked frontal headache and photophobia. Pains in the back and down the legs followed, but no epigastric pain or tenderness; vomiting set in the following day, at first bilious, but gradually becoming quite black in character.

" He noticed that his gums bled about the same time.

' His motions were of a dark colour, becoming almost quite black. His urine soon became of a light red colour, but never dark red or black

' The hot condition of his skin lasted until the day before he was discharged, that is six days, and remained constant during this period

' No record of jaundice, temperature, pulse, examination of blood or urine could be found.

" No further details of case could be ascertained from the patient himself.

" Patient was discharged cured on the 12th September, 1913."

These cases at Bole are of special interest, as they may illustrate how the disease is kept in being. If Dr. Lundie had not been infected, it is certain that nothing would have been heard of the attacks from which the two native policemen suffered in the previous September. Both these earlier cases in natives were, in the opinion of the Commission, "Probably Yellow Fever," of the type which is not uncommonly met with in such patients.

. Vol. II., ɔ. 696. se No. 4).

The following case in a native also occurred at Bole, in 1913:—

CASE 1.—*Edi, Hausa.—Native* (*Unknown*).

" *Movement of patient.*—It has proved somewhat difficult to obtain definite information concerning the movements of this patient. He was said to have been in Bole about seven, and at most ten, days ere his death, and had come from Kintampo, where he had resided for some time. In Bole his movements had been quite obscure, sometimes the patient having passed the night in one hut and moving to some other place the following night.

" Patient first attended hospital on 8th December, 1913, as an out-patient, and complained of constipation (' No fit go latrine '), anorexia, and epigastric pains, which, on questioning him, seemed to be of a dyspeptic nature.

"Pulse and temperature were normal, and at no time had he suffered from pains in the head or diarrhœa. There was a complete absence of photophobia, bleeding from buccal mucous membrane, and any icteric tinging of the conjunctivæ. Mist. alba was prescribed, and he was told to come to hospital the following morning, 9th December, 1913. Whilst in the dispensary he vomited about one-and-a-half ounces of fluid, which on examination proved to be of simple gastric origin. According to his own statement he had never vomited before this date.

"From the foregoing symptoms, and also the examination of the patient, there was nothing to make one even suspicious that it might be Yellow Fever, and I had nothing to justify me in detaining him or regarding him as such.

"The following morning, 9th December, he did not appear at hospital, and on the morning of 10th December I was informed by the dispenser that the patient who had visited me on the morning of 8th December was very ill and unable to come to hospital.

"I had the patient at once brought into hospital in my hammock, and the following is a Report on his condition when admitted:—

"Patient was in a moribund condition; there was some clotted blood on the lips, and on examination the gums were oozing freely, and the conjunctival reflex was gone. The scleras were of a well-marked icteric tinge and injected.

"Axillary temperature was 101·4° Fahr., and the pulse imperceptible. About half an hour after admission to hospital the patient vomited about one ounce of fluid, black in colour, and containing blood which had evidently been acted upon by the gastric juice.

"The patient never recovered from his comatose condition, and died about one-and-a-half hours after being admitted to hospital.

"The axillary temperature was taken about fifteen minutes after death, and registered 104·6° Fahr. The above symptoms being rather suggestive of Yellow Fever, and sanction to perform a post-mortem having been obtained, an autopsy was performed soon after death.

Post-mortem.

"The body is that of a young man whose bodily nutrition is fair. The lips and oral mucous membranes are covered with clotted blood

"The scleræ are of a marked yellow colour.

"Post-mortem rigidity present.

"On cutting through the dark epidermis and reaching the cutis vera, it is found to be of a lemon colour. On opening the abdomen the abdominal visceræ are injected and of a very faint lemon colour.

"The great omentum was very markedly congested.

"*Thorax.*—On opening through, the pericardical sac is found to contain about half an ounce of pale straw-coloured pericardical fluid.

"*Heart.*—The heart is pale in colour, normal in size, and flabby in consistence. On section the heart muscle is pale in appearance and shows at one or two points petechial hæmorrhages.

"Fatty degeneration is also present.

"*Lungs.*—The lungs are slightly larger than normal, and are markedly congested.

"On section they present a congested appearance, slightly emphysematous, and numerous enlarged peribronchial glands. The bronchi contain a small amount of mucoid secretion.

"*Parietal pleuræ.*—The parietal pleuræ have numerous small subparietal hæmorrhages.

"*Liver.*—The liver is larger than normal.

"Glisson's capsule somewhat adherent, and here and there deeply injected. The walls of the gall bladder show considerable hypertrophy, and the bladder itself contains about two drachms of inspissated bile. No biliary calculi present.

"On section the liver is pale in appearance, friable, and the hepatic cells are swollen.

"*Spleen.*—This organ is three times the normal in size, of a dark slate colour, and very friable. On section it is markedly congested and very friable.

"*Kidneys.*—Both kidneys are of normal size.

"Capsules strip easily. On section they present a congested appearance, especially marked in the pyramids.

"*Gastro-intestinal tract.*—The stomach is markedly congested. On opening into the stomach it is found to contain about two ounces of fluid, dark in colour, and containing digested blood.

"The rugæ of the stomach are markedly injected, and swollen.

"The mucosa is swollen, injected, and coated with a thin semi-gelatinous film, to which adheres semi-digested blood. The above pathological condition is general in this viscus, but more marked towards the pylorus.

"*Intestines.*—The duodenum presents the same pathological condition as the stomach, and the contents are mingled with blood.

"*Small intestine.*—The small intestine is injected, but to a lesser degree than that found in the stomach and duodenum. The contents here are darker in colour, and contain blood.

"*Large intestine.*—There is nothing pathologically worthy of note to be found in the large intestine.

"The contents here are quite black and characteristic of melæna. No other pathological lesion sufficient to cause death was found.

"*Urine.*—The bladder being empty no urine could be obtained for analysis.

"*Blood.*—Thick and thin blood smears were taken.

"*Summary.*—From the symptoms of this case and the pathological lesions found post-mortem. I regard this case as having been one of Yellow Fever.

"Medical Officer, Bole."

(*f*) KINTAMPO.

1913.

Kintampo is situated in Northern Ashanti, lying 8° 3′ N., 1° 41′ W.

The patient was a European official in his fourth tour of service. He landed at Seccondee on 23rd September, 1913, and travelled viâ Coomassie, leaving that town on 2nd October. He slept for the first three nights in native houses, in the villages between Coomassie and Chichewera, and the remaining three nights he slept in the rest-houses for Europeans, which are situated some little distance away from the villages. He arrived at Kintampo on October 8th, and was taken ill on October 16th. He died from Yellow Fever on October 19th.

(*g*) TUMU.

1913.

Tumu is a town in the North Western District of the Northern Territories of the Gold Coast. It lies 9° 54′ N., 1° 58′ W., and is only some eight miles from the northern boundary. The patient was the District Commissioner, Northern Territories; he was taken ill on 15th November, 1913, and died from Yellow Fever on November 22nd.

ANALYSIS OF SPORADIC CASES IN 1914.

(III.) SIERRA LEONE.

BOIA.

1914.

This case was classified by a majority of the Commission as one of "Yellow Fever," the others were disposed to class it under the heading "Probable."

The patient was a European, æt. 32, on his third year of service in Sierra Leone. He was taken ill on March 9th, 1914, at Boia, a station on the main line of railway at its junction with the branch line to Makump, distant about 60 miles from Freetown. Boia contains five bungalows for Europeans, a mud built rest-house and a reservation for railway employees and labourers; about eight Europeans are stationed there. The patient was removed to the Nursing Home at Freetown on March 13th and recovered after a moderately severe attack of Yellow Fever, which is fully described in Appendix D., page 574 (I.R., Vol. II.).

The patient had not spent a night away from Boia for some months previous to his illness, and his duties did not carry him up or down the line for any distance. No other cases occurred amongst the Europeans, and no suspicious cases of fever were found amongst the sick natives of the surrounding villages, who were specially sent to Boia for examination during the visit of the Investigator appointed to report upon the case in question. It is of interest to note that the report states that not a single *Culicine* larva was discovered or a mosquito of any kind seen in the villages within easy reach of Boia, although a few *Anopheline* larvæ were found in a stream of running water in a valley below the railway.

The case of Yellow Fever occurred in a double bungalow occupied by the fitter and foreman platelayer on the railway. The mosquito nets in the house were in holes and quite unfit for use. The native reservation at Boia is placed at about 800 yards from the nearest European bungalow.

It may be noted as a point of clinical and pathological interest in connection with this case that granular casts stained yellow were present in the urine on six examinations. The importance of this sign is mentioned in the chapter on the "Diagnosis of Yellow Fever," by Dr. Hamilton P. Jones in Augustin's "History of Yellow Fever" (page 1,157), and the attention of Investigators had been specially directed to it by the Commission.

This case is another example of the difficulty experienced in discovering the source of infection in sporadic cases occurring in the interior of the country.

(IV) GOLD COAST.

(*a*) QUITTAH.

1914.

Amongst the fever cases investigated during the months of March and April, 1914, by Dr. G. E. H. Le Fanu there are some of special interest.

The history of Quittah in relation to Yellow Fever, as known at the date of the Second Report of the Commission, is as follows (*vide* Second Report, page 70, *et seq.*):—

"1888.

"There was one case of sporadic yellow fever. Deaths also occurred from 'Ardent Remittent Fever.'"

"1893.

"'Bilious remittent fever' was general in the towns on the Gold Coast.

"The incidence of disease at Quittah was so excessive that among the community there was a state which I venture to call 'fever panic.'"

"1894.

"Three Europeans ill with malarial fever, one of the so-called bilious, the other of the 'remittent type.' On the basis of classification adopted by the Commission a case which occurred at Quittah in this year is classified as 'Yellow Fever.'"

From the above it is clear that at the dates mentioned Quittah was an endemic focus of Yellow Fever.

April, 1914.

The case No. 26 (I.R., Vol. II., page 589) has been classified by the Commission as one of Yellow Fever after receiving a report from Dr. A. C. Stevenson of the Wellcome Research Bureau.

The patient was a native, female, aged 28, who died in Hospital at Quittah on April 6th, 1914, of Yellow Fever, after an illness lasting nine days.

No history was obtained of the patient's movements prior to the illness. She led an irregular life and probably lived in Quittah.

No other cases occurred at the time.

May, 1914.

In the following case the Commission were divided in opinion:—

Case of Kpesu.

Commentary by the Commission.

(1) The onset was very sudden, with severe rigor, pains and frontal headache.

(2) A remission occurred on the fourth day, when there was marked epigastric tenderness, considerable albuminuria and jaundice.

(3) Prostration is described as "marked" on the following day. Faget's sign was present: the pulse rate having fallen from 140 to 76.

(4) Granular casts were found in the urine on the fourth and sixth days.

(5) After a period of gradual improvement, during which no quinine was given, and no malarial parasites were found in the blood, the patient recovered, and was discharged from hospital.

(6) Two days later, May 30th (*i.e.*, the eleventh day since the onset), the patient returned, stating that he felt cold and ill "and that he got ill." The spleen was now enlarged, and the blood was found to contain tertian parasites. The temperature was 100° F. and the pulse 100. No quinine was taken until prescribed for the malarial attack on May 30th.

(7) The Medical Officer reporting on the case said:—"Three pigmented leucocytes were found in four thick films on 23rd and 24th May, after examination totalling one and a half hours. I attach no diagnostic importance."

(8) The above facts are certainly consistent with a diagnosis of mild Yellow Fever in a native already the subject of malarial infection.

June 1914.

In the following case the Commission were divided in opinion as to the classification:—

Case of Kofie.

Commentary by the Commission.

(1) The onset was sudden, with severe rigor, violent headache and pains in the loins.

(2) There was marked prostration; the eyes were strongly injected, fiery and red; there was violent frontal headache and the urine was scanty; albuminuria was present. Jaundice and epigastric tenderness were absent on admission; both appeared later.

(3) Faget's sign was marked. The pulse fell from 102 to 56.

(4) The albumen gradually disappeared from the urine.

(5) A stool contained eggs of *Ascaris lumbricoides* at a period of the illness when the temperature was 103° F. or 102° F. and the pulse 92 to 83.

(6) No parasites or pigment were found in the peripheral blood.

(7) The above symptoms are consistent with the diagnosis of a moderately severe attack of Yellow Fever in a native.

(b) SALTPOND.

May, 1914.

The following case was classified by a majority of the Commission as "Probable Yellow Fever."

"Clinical notes on case of Mr. H. B., six months on Coast, first time abroad, age 23 years, assistant, Basel Mission Factory, Saltpond.

"I was called to see patient at 11.30 a.m. on the 27th May; he had been ill since the morning of the 25th May, and that his temperature had been over 39 centigrade on both days, he had passed 12 dark watery motions, and just before my arrival had vomited a little greenish fluid.

"During the two days he had taken 12 grains of powdered quinine.

"29th May. On examination:—

"Face flushed, frontal and occipital headache, tongue clean, no liver or abdominal tenderness, had slept badly. Temperature 101°, pulse 77.

"Ordered liquid quinine, 10 grains, Aspirin 10 grains, took blood smears.

"6 p.m. Temperature 101°, pulse 75, had vomited once after taking some soup. Skin moist. Urine clear, light coloured, Sp. gr. 1030, acid, no albumen. Ordered quinine 10 grains to be given in the morning. No parasites found in blood.

"30th May:—

"8 a.m. Temperature 101°, pulse 72, slept badly. Bowels moved once, light coloured, no vomiting, headache, urine—no albumen.

"12 o'clock. Temperature 101·4°, pulse 70. Bowels opened, loose dark motion. Gave quinine 7 grains hypodermically.

"6 p.m. Temperature 102·6°, pulse 74. Conjunctivæ yellow. Complained of pains in stomach. Nausea—felt tired. Ordered Sternberg's mixture hourly. Hot pack over stomach.

"31st May:—

"1 a.m. Temperature 102·4°, pulse 70. Restless. Taking mixture well.

"6 a.m. Temperature 102°, pulse 68. Skin and conjunctivæ lemon coloured, nausea, no vomiting, has passed no urine for 12 hours. Slept badly. Bowels opened once, liquid dark coloured. Took brandy 1 ounce twice.

"10 a.m. No change. Temperature 102°, pulse 68.

"2 p.m. Passed urine 4 ounces, light coloured, heavy with albumen. Hot pack to loins, very restless.

"6 p.m. Temperature 101·2°, pulse 66. Urine 3 ounces.

"10 p.m. Temperature 101·4°, pulse 66. Slept a little.

" 1st June :—

" 2 a.m. Temperature 100°, pulse 64.

" 6 a.m. Temperature 100·4°, pulse 68. Slept badly, restless, took fluids well. Champagne 2 ounces.

" 10 a.m. Very yellow. Temperature 100·6°, pulse 66. Said he felt well.

" 2 p.m. No urine passed, looked bad. Breath sounds sighing. Hot pack continued.

" 6 p.m. Temperature 100·4°, pulse 60. Urine 8 ounces. Albumen nearly solid. Complained of discomfort about the stomach, some tenderness.

" 10 p.m. Temperature 100·4°, pulse 64. Felt tired.

" 2nd June :—

" 2 a.m. Asleep.

" 6 a.m. Urine, albumen heavy, slept for three hours in the night. Temperature 100°, pulse 66.

" 12 o'clock. Temperature 100°, pulse 64. Not inclined to take nourishment. Taking Sternberg's fairly well, very yellow.

" 3 p.m. Temperature 100°, pulse 64. Very dull.

" 6 p.m. Had two hours' sleep.

" 10 p.m. Passed urine 10 ounces, very dark. Temperature 100°, pulse 60.

" 3rd June :—

" 3 a.m. Temperature 99·4°. Had some sleep.

" 6 a.m. Temperature 99°, pulse 64. Slept.

" 10.30 a.m. Urine 14 ounces, very dark, bile pigment present. Albumen heavy.

" 2 p.m. Slept; felt better. Temperature 90·4°, pulse 66. Taking more liquids.

" 6 p.m. Temperature 98·6°, pulse 62. Had two hours' sleep. Passed urine, vomited clear fluid at 5.30.

" 10 p.m. Bowels opened. Stool light coloured.

" 4th June :—

" 2 a.m. Temperature 98°, pulse 64.

" 6 a.m. Temperature 98°, pulse —. Slept well.

" 10 p.m. Temperature 98° all day, pulse 64. Took nourishment well. Passed 12 ounces urine, bile pigment. Albumen less, still heavy.

" 5th June :—

" 7 a.m. Temperature 99°, pulse 60. Slept well.

" 12 o'clock. Temperature 99·4°, pulse 62. Passed urine, albumen.

" 6 p.m. Temperature 100°, pulse 62. Says he feels well. Passed urine, albumen.

" 6th June :—

" 6.30 a.m. Temperature 100°, pulse 64. Had a good night.

" 10.30 a.m. Temperature 99°, pulse 62. Albumen less in urine, bile pigment present, urine increasing in quantity.

"3 p.m. Temperature 98·4°, pulse 74. Passed urine; taking liquids largely. Brand's beef juice, Benger's food in small quantities.

"6 p.m. Temperature 98°, pulse 64.

"7th June:—

"6.30 a.m Good night. Passed 26 ounces urine, dark in colour, no albumen. Still jaundiced. Temperature 80°, pulse 62.

"3 o'clock. Comfortable.

"6 p.m. Temperature 98°, pulse 66.

"8th June:—

"8 a.m. Temperature 98·4°, pulse 68. Slept well. Bowels open. Urine 23 ounces, no albumen."

(*c*) TAMALE.

1914.

Tamale, which lies 9° 22′ 30″ N., 0° 51′ W., is a town in the Southern District of the Northern Territories of the Gold Coast. The patient was a native of Calabar, and had been working in the Northern Territories for some time. He had been ill about three days when seen on August 20th at Tamale, where he had gone for treatment.

The Commission were divided as to the classification of the case.

Commentary.

The points of interest in this case are:—

(1) The swelling of the submaxillary glands. These glands and the parotid have been noted as enlarged in a small percentage of cases of yellow fever.

(2) Albumen appeared in the urine on the fourth day, increased markedly on the fifth, diminished on the sixth and disappeared on the seventh day.

(3) Faget's sign was marked; the pulse falling to 40 and rising again, but only to 62.

(4) Absence of Malaria parasites.

(5) Marked headache and photophobia.

On December 3rd, 1914, two other cases of Yellow Fever were reported from Tamale.

The records of these cases have not reached the Commission.

(*d*) BOLE.

May, 1914.

The patient was a native boy, æt. 11 years, who was taken ill on April 30th, 1914, and died in Hospital at Bole of Yellow Fever on May 4th. A post-mortem examination was made and characteristic lesions were found.

(c) AXIM.

1914.

Axim is situated on the seaboard of the Gold Coast, and lies 4° 52′ N., 1° 13′ W.

The following fatal case occurred on July 19th, 1914. The patient was Mr. C., a European official.

In this case, locally diagnosed as Yellow Fever, the Commission were divided in opinion.

"MEDICAL REPORT ON THE ILLNESS AND DEATH OF MR. C.

"On the forenoon of the 13th I was called in to see Mr. C., and found him in a rather collapsed condition, with pale, pinched features and conjunctivæ markedly injected. He was vomiting a considerable amount of bilious matter. He had slight headache, slight tenderness over the epigastrium, slight enlargement of the liver, but no tenderness, no tenderness over the gall-bladder, and no tenderness over the rest of the abdomen or back. The tongue was coated with a white fur, and he was badly constipated. His temperature was 99°, pulse 84.

"He informed me that he had had a slight go of fever on Saturday, but had taken some quinine and felt all right in the morning. On Monday he went down to the office feeling rather out of sorts, and about 10 a.m. had a rigor which lasted for one hour, when he began to vomit. The vomit at first was sour-tasting liquid containing half-digested food, then became green in nature.

"He spent a very bad night, vomiting all the time, and passed seven or eight motions.

"On the 14th he became jaundiced and the conjunctivæ quite green. The tongue was also coated with a green fur. He complained of no pains anywhere. Temperature 100°, pulse 94. He was admitted to hospital at once. There were no signs of skin rash, hæmorrhages, or bleeding from the gums now or any time during the illness. He continued vomiting all day a greenish liquid with black masses in it and mucus, and could keep nothing in his stomach. He also passed three motions which were very black and soft in nature and also green slimy fluid. No urine was passed separate to the motions, so I was unable to test it.

"His temperature was now 102°, pulse 94, and remained so all day. He had an injection of morphia at 5 p.m. and slept from 6 p.m. to 5 a.m. next morning.

"15th.—His temperature had now fallen to 98°, pulse 84. He continued much the same all day, continually vomiting, still very jaundiced, passed no urine. Microscopic examination failed to show any signs of malarial parasites in the blood.

"16th.—Patient had a fairly good night, and was looking much better, the icterus much reduced, vomiting much reduced and no black material in it. Temperature 97°, pulse 80. Passed no urine all day. He was able to take a little chicken broth and retained it.

"17th.—Passed fairly good night; slept from 11 p.m. to 5 a.m. Temperature 97·4°, pulse 80. He had very slight vomiting. No urine passed.

"18th.—Passed very good night. Temperature 98·4, pulse 80. He passed one motion, which was very liquid and brown in colour, but not smelling badly. No urine was passed. He was much brighter himself, but he wandered at times, and his mind seemed to be a blank at times. His temperature in the evening was 98°, but his pulse had increased to 106. He slept till 4 a.m., when his temperature had risen to 100°, pulse 110, and he had uræmic convulsions. He passed out of these into a state of coma and continued in this condition till 7.30 a.m., when he expired."

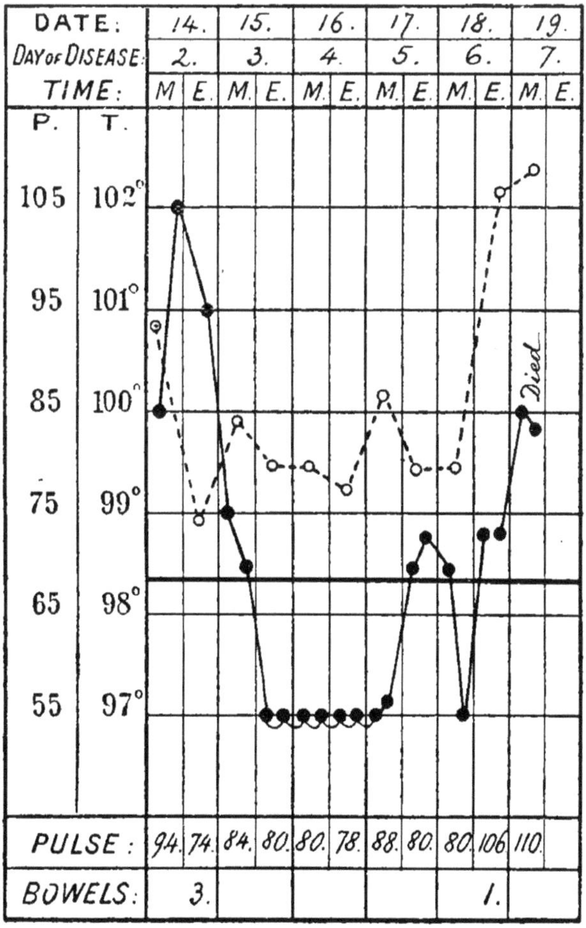

DATE:	14.		15.		16.		17.		18.		19.	
DAY OF DISEASE:	2.		3.		4.		5.		6.		7.	
TIME:	M	E.	M.	E.	M.	E.	M.	E.	M.	E.	M.	E.
PULSE:	94.	74.	84.	80.	80.	78.	88.	80.	80.	106	110.	
BOWELS:	3.								1.			

Died

P.	T.
105	102°
95	101°
85	100°
75	99°
65	98°
55	97°

"*Treatment.*—Champagne was the only liquid he could keep down. He was given this in equal quantities of soda water.

"Mag. Sulp., Bismuth, and Ac. Hydrocyan. dil. were given the first day, but he could not keep them down. Calomel was tried and Ac. Nit. Hydrochlor. dil. was tried when he came into hospital, with same result. He was then put on Sternberg's solution, 1½ ounces hourly, and morphia to stop the excessive vomiting. Cocaine was tried first with *nil* results.

"The anuria was treated with hot fomentations, salines, blistering, hot packs, and pilocarpine, but with no response.

"*Post-mortem.*—Lungs were very pale and anæmic, otherwise normal. Heart normal.

"Stomach: mucosa congested and bile-stained; fluid contained bile pigment and albumen and a lot of debris.

"Pylorus and upper part of jejunum was also congested.

"Spleen slightly enlarged and congested.

"Liver slightly enlarged and congested, and stained with bile. Gall-bladder full of semi-liquid bile.

"Kidney enlarged, much congested, and of a mottled grey appearance. Capsule not adherent. Tubules standing out very prominent. Bladder small and empty.

"Medical Officer."

Commentary.

(1) This patient's history sheet shows that he had an attack of malarial fever on 28th October, 1911, and was discharged recovered on 31st October.

(2) He stated that "he had an attack like this twelve years ago in British Guiana." It appears that a patient who has suffered from Malaria and is subsequently attacked by Yellow Fever is usually able to differentiate between the two illnesses.

(3) The onset appears to have been sudden and severe, as he was "rather collapsed with pale pinched features and conjunctivæ markedly injected."

(4) The vomiting was severe and consisted of a greenish liquid with black masses in it. The stools were "very black."

(5) There was a marked remission in the symptoms on the fourth day.

(6) Death was due to uræmia with suppression of urine and convulsions.

(7) No malarial parasites were found in the blood.

The foregoing symptoms are consistent with a diagnosis of Yellow Fever, which was the cause given on the certificate of death.

(*f*) SOMANYA.

Somanya is about 52 miles slightly north-east from Accra, with which it is connected by a motor road. It has a population of four European merchants and about 4,000 natives. There is no segregation for Europeans, and they live in the centre of the town near the market-place.

In the following case, locally diagnosed as Yellow Fever, the Commission were divided in opinion:—

"REPORT ON ILLNESS AND DEATH OF E. H. H., SOMANYA.

"1. Mr. E. H. H. has been five-and-a-half years on the West Coast.

"In November of last year (1913) he was treated for pleuro-pneumonia, and was confined to bed for ten days.

"In December of the same year (1913) he developed phlebitis, and was invalided home in February, 1914.

"He came back to the Coast in May, 1914, and again developed phlebitis. In July he was able to walk about quite fit until I saw him in his last illness.

"2. On the 13th of August, 1914, I was called to attend Mr. H., who was suffering from what he termed bilious vomiting and persistent hiccup.

"3. On examination I found the tongue was furred and the temperature was subnormal, 96·5°, and his pulse 99, urine contained trace of albumen.

"4. His skin and conjunctivæ showed slight icterus.

"5. Over the epigastrium he complained of very severe pain which on palpation seemed to be localized over the region of the gall bladder.

"He also complained of constipation, but put this down to the fact that he had nothing to eat for the previous three days, as he was very liverish.

"6. The vomit was on the 15th composed of mucus, but he informed me previous to my visit the vomit contained bile.

"7. His blood on microscopic examination showed no abnormal changes.

"8. I again visited him on the morning of the 16th, and found that the epigastric pain was more pronounced, as also was the hiccup.

"The vomit remained clear and mucoid in character.

"9. The temperature remained subnormal, 95°, and the pulse was 101. In the evening of the same day, about seven o'clock, the vomit was composed of a brownish grumous material, which gave the reaction for blood.

"10. This vomit persisted during the night at intervals of about two hours.

"He died at 4.30 on the morning of the 16th.

"*Treatment.*—Hot fomentations were applied to the epigastrium. Calomel grains iii. were given, and a mixture was prescribed for the vomiting.

Post-mortem Appearances.—Post-mortem rigidity set in very quickly; all the dependent parts, back of neck, and all posterior part of body showed marked ecchymoses.

"Black, inky fluid was coming out of the mouth.

"The skin showed slight yellow tinge.

"*The Lungs.*—The right lung showed old-standing cavity at base with pleural adhesions. The left lung showed small pea-like foci of necrosis scattered throughout. Both lungs were congested.

"*Heart.*—The heart showed small punctiform hæmorrhage, otherwise normal.

"*Liver.*—The liver was normal in size, and of a pale brownish colour. The gall bladder contained a small quantity of bile.

"*Stomach.*—The stomach contained black, inky fluid. The stomach wall was inflamed, and showed small punctiform hæmorrhages. The small intestines were uniformly of a black colour and contained inky fluid. The intestinal wall and mesentery of small intestine were very friable. The large intestine was not so much affected as the small. There were punctiform hæmorrhages throughout.

"The kidneys were congested.

"The bladder was normal.

"The urine contained albumen.

"The spleen was normal in size, and slightly congested.

"*Diagnosis.*—Yellow fever.

"Medical Officer,
"Akuse."

There were no further cases.

(V.) NIGERIA--NORTHERN PROVINCES.

JEBBA.

1914.

Up to the date of the occurrence of the following case, Yellow Fever had not been known in Northern Nigeria. The case was classified by the Commission as "Probable Yellow Fever." The patient was employed on the Nigerian Railway. Death took place on the train between Jebba and Zungeru. The facts of the case, so far as known, are as follows. At the inquest the Medical Officer of the district stated:—

"On Saturday, 10th July, I received a wire at 8 a.m. from Mr. W, at Jebba Island, asking me to come up and see one of his assistants who was having continuous fever. I caught a light engine going to Jebba, and arrived Jebba about noon. As soon as possible I crossed the river and saw the patient; he was in a grass hut with cement floor. I examined him and found his temperature 105·2° and pulse 102 fairly strong, furred tongue, and had been vomiting, usual in malarial fever. I gave the patient five grains calomel and five grains phenacetin and hot drinks; he seemed in fairly good condition, his pulse gave me no anxiety. I stayed with him for two hours; I then went to see another patient at Jebba South, Driver M, N.R., who had a temperature over 105°. Before leaving I gave instructions to Mr. W.'s assistant to look after the patient with directions. I returned at 6 p.m. when I found Driver M.'s temperature falling; I found Mr. D.'s temperature had dropped to 103·2°, his pulse was quick but fairly strong; during the night I stayed with the patient, seeing him frequently, his pulse remained about 103 all night, his urine was normal and there were no physical signs pointing either to heart failure or blackwater fever. As I had another serious case at Jebba South I found it absolutely impossible to give the attention I considered necessary to both patients. I therefore asked Mr. W. to have Mr. D. taken to Zungeru Hospital, which, in my opinion, was the best thing to do for the patient, and to be sent in charge of Mr. W.'s assistant, to whom I gave full instructions. I proceeded to Jebba South to see Driver M., and was informed by telephone message that the patient had left at 10.30. At about noon, Mr. W. arrived and informed me that the patient had not left. I immediately went to the island and saw the patient; his temperature was 103° and fairly quick pulse; the patient seemed quite comfortable, and at 2 p.m. I saw him into the train with Mr. W.'s assistant when they left for Zungeru."

The report on the post-mortem examination is as follows:—

"The post-mortem examination was made on the morning of 13th July, about seven hours after death had occurred.

"The deceased died on the train during transit from Jebba to Zungeru. History given by a non-medical man was of high fever for three days, followed by collapse with apparent suppression of urine, and in the last few hours with black vomit.

"*Appearance.*—Post-mortem lividity was well marked. The conjunctivæ were distinctly yellow.

"*Thorax.*—Lungs congested but containing air: right, 11½ oz.; left, 10 oz. Heart rather flabby, otherwise normal. Weight, 11 oz.

"*Abdomen.*—No free fluid present. Stomach contained a small quantity of thin fluid black with altered blood. Mucous membrane of stomach, duodenum, and first part of jejunum showed numerous small petechial hæmorrhages. The remaining part of the intestine showed nothing abnormal. Liver was distinctly yellow in colour. It was dry, had retained its shape, and was of fairly firm consistency; weight, 2 lbs. 10½ oz. Spleen was enlarged and rather soft. It was distinctly pigmented; weight, 7½ oz. Kidneys showed some congestion, but little, if any, comparative swelling of the cortex; right, 5 oz.; left, 5½ oz. Bladder contained no urine.

"*Brain.*—Some congestion of meninges. No malarial pigmentation of capillaries.

"*Blood examination* (from jugular vein).—Corpuscles rather degenerated, and staining therefore irregular. Fairly numerous subtertian malaria parasites were present.

"*Spleen smear.*—Pigment in spleen cells, but not in excessive quantity. Some malaria parasites were recognizable in the erythrocytes.

"In view of the comparatively mild malarial infection present, the jaundice, the condition of stomach, liver and kidneys, and the absence of urine from the bladder, the post-mortem findings decidedly suggest that *death was due to Yellow Fever.* Italics in original.

"Acting Senior Medical Officer.

"14th July, 1914."

The results of the microscopical examination of the tissues were as follows:—

"*Spleen.*—Congested.

"*Liver.*—Congestion. Outline of lobules lost. Great destruction of hepatic cells and marked fatty degeneration.

"*Kidneys.*—Glomerular tufts swollen and showing hæmorrhages. Vessels generally engorged. Marked necrosis and desquamation of lining cells of all the tubules. Lumen of tubules filled with débris.

"MINUTE BY THE DIRECTOR OF MEDICAL AND SANITARY SERVICES.

"C.S.

"There is no doubt in my mind that Mr. D. died of Yellow Fever.

"Director Medical Service.

"22nd July, 1914."

(VI.) NIGERIA.—SOUTHERN PROVINCES.

(*a*) EBUTE-METTA (LAGOS).

1914.

28. In the following case the Commission were divided in opinion:—

"REPORT.—YELLOW FEVER. L. 128.

"Name: A. O'C.

"Sex: Male.

"Age: 27 years.

"Nationality: British.

"Date of admission: 8th March, 1914.

"Date of discharge: 20th March, 1914.

"Diagnosis: Yellow Fever.

"Result: Recovery.

"*History.*—Patient has only been out for three weeks of his first tour of service in Nigeria. Previous to coming to Lagos, he had been for three months in Sierra Leone.

"He states that he first got ill on the 5th March with a severe frontal headache, followed by rigors and pyrexia. He also had severe pains in the back and extremities. Temperature was raised and was 105 that night. He was seen by the Medical Officer at Ebute-Metta and treated. Next day, the 6th, he was much the same, with severe headache and temperature of 104°. On the 7th, his temperature was still high and he noticed that his urine was diminished, and on examination, was found to contain albumen. He was sent into hospital on the 8th and admitted at 1 p.m.

" Patient states that he had been taking quinine regularly during the illness, but previous to that very irregularly. Vomiting was present on the 6th, with epigastric pain and discomfort, and on the 7th he had no vomiting but nausea was distressing.

" *On admission.*—Patient seemed in distress. Face was flushed. Eyes shining. Conjunctivæ injected and red. Pain in the eyes also present. Temperature was 103·8°, pulse rate 88. Complained of severe frontal headache and pains in the back and extremities.

" *Alimentary System.*—Tongue was pointed with furred dorsum and red tip and edges. Bowels have been constipated. Vomiting had been present at the commencement of the illness, but nausea is now present. Epigastric pain and discomfort present. Liver and spleen are both normal, no tenderness on palpation.

" *Circulatory System.*—Heart sounds are normal. Pulse rate is 88.

" *Respiratory System.*—Lungs were normal. Respirations were 22.

" *Urinary System.*—Urine is diminished in quantity and high coloured. On examination: Acid reaction. Sp. gr. 1025. Albumen present. Tube casts also present.

" *Blood examination.*—Few subtertian malaria parasites present. Leucopenia present. Differential count: Polymorph., 54·8 per cent.; lymphocyte, 24·8 per cent.; mononuclear, 16·2 per cent.; transitional, 4 per cent.; mast cells, 2 per cent.

" 8 p.m. Temperature was 102·6°, pulse rate 100.

" 9th March.—Patient had a fair night, headache was severe, also pains in the back and extremities. Temperature at 8 a.m. was 101°. Bowels were opened after the calomel. Urine was diminished, and only three ozs. passed in the 12 hours. Very high coloured and containing albumen. Acid reaction. Sp. gr. 1020. Epigastric pain and discomfort still present.

" 10th March.—Patient had a better night. Headache and loin pains not so severe. Passed no urine at all during the past 24 hours. Passed about one oz. at 10 p.m. Albumen present. Sp. gr. 1030. Acid reaction. Headache was increased towards the afternoon. Temperature at 8 a.m. was 99·4°, pulse rate 76, and at 8 p.m. it was the same, with a pulse rate of 64. Scleræ were tinged with yellow.

" 11th March.—Patient had a good night and slept well. Urine passed but still diminished. Albumen present. Acid reaction. Sp. gr. 1025. Scleræ are yellow. Bowels opened. Headache and loin pains have gone. Slight epigastric discomfort still present. Temperature at 8 a.m. was 99°, pulse rate 64, and at 8 p.m. 98·4°, with pulse of 54.

" 12th March.—Patient had a good night and feels very much better. Scleræ are very yellow. Urine has increased in quantity. On examination is acid in reaction. Sp. gr. 1030. No albumen present. Bile has now appeared. Appetite is improving. Temperature at 8 a.m. 97·4°, pulse rate 54, and at 8 p.m. 98·4°, with pulse of 60.

"13th March.—Patient feeling very much better. Had a good night. Appetite improved. Bowels opened. Urine normal and increased in amount. Jaundice well marked. Temperature normal, pulse still slow. Patient continued to do well. Jaundice disappeared on the 18th, and the patient was discharged cured on the 20th March."

The blood count was as follows:—

	8th March. Subtertian rings.	9th March. Subtertian rings.	10th March. 0
Polymorphonuclears	62·2 per cent.	54·8 per cent.	43·8 per cent.
Lymphocytes ...	23·0 ,,	24·4 ,,	28·2 ,,
Mononuclears ...	12·0 ,,	16·2 ,,	20·8 ,,
Eosinophiles ...	0·2 ,,	— ,,	1·4 ,,
Transitionals ...	2·2 ,,	4·0 ,,	5·8 ,,
Mast cells	0·4 ,,	0·2 ,,	—

(*b*) CALABAR.

133. The following case, diagnosed locally as Yellow Fever, occurred on the s.s. "Yola," on April 22nd, 1914. The details are incomplete, and the Commission were divided in opinion as to its nature.

The patient was a Russian sailor, æt. 27.

The following report contains all that is known of the case:—

"REPORT ON A CASE OF YELLOW FEVER OCCURRING AT CALABAR ON S.S. 'YOLA.'

"I boarded s.s. 'Yola' on the 25th April, 1914, and then saw F. Tomsen, A.B. He was then apparently suffering from malarial fever, having a temperature of 101°, a pulse of 90, no epigastric pain or any vomiting or jaundice. He had been feverish since the 22nd April, 1914. He subsequently died at 2.30 p.m. on the 25th April, 1914, but his death was not reported to me until about 9 a.m. on the 26th April, 1914. I went on board the s.s. 'Yola' again and elicited the fact that when Tomsen died his temperature was 109° The history I then obtained was as follows:—

"22nd April, 1914. Headache. Temperature 105° in morning.
Temperature 101° ,, evening.

"23rd April, 1914. Temperature 98·4° in morning.
Temperature 104° ,, evening.

"24th April, 1914. Temperature 98·4° ,, morning.
Temperature 98·4° ,, evening.

"25th April, 1914. Temperature 98·4° in morning, 6 a.m.
Temperature 101° at 10 a.m.
Temperature 105° ,, 12 noon.
Temperature 108° ,, 1.30 p.m.
Temperature 109° ,, 2.30 p.m.
with convulsions and death.

"The body was already coffined at 10 a.m., 26th April, 1914. I had the coffin opened and found the body in a rapidly advancing stage of decomposition, but showing purplish blotches on chest and penis. I had the body removed to the mortuary, where I made a post-mortem examination; post-mortem report attached.

"Medical Officer.

"*Post-mortem Report.*

"Body that of a male, bloated, and decomposition advanced. Purple staining on chest and neck and slightly of scrotum and penis, bloody fluid oozing from mouth. Abdomen was opened; stomach removed, and on opening found to be filled with black coffee-ground material. Mucous membrane intensely injected. Liver enlarged, soft, does not show to naked eye any fatty change.

"Spleen large and very friable and engorged.

"Kidneys both large, and show small petechiæ under capsule and also white patches.

"Bladder contained a small amount of cloudy urine, and on examination was found to contain albumen.

"Stomach and contents, portions of liver, spleen, and kidneys removed, and smears taken of liver, kidney, and spleen; specimens sent to Medical Research Institute for report.

"Medical Officer."

(c) BURUTU.

1914.

Burutu is situated about five miles up-river from Forcados in the Warri Province of the Southern Provinces of Nigeria, and was at one time the transport station for the Northern Nigeria Government. The Niger Company has a large shipping depôt, together with extensive engineering shops there, and a slipway which is capable of taking fairly large craft. Usually there are about 20 Europeans at Burutu. The native population is about 1,480. Burutu lies 5° 19′ N., 5° 34′ E.

ON BOARD SS. "ASHANTI."—OCTOBER, 1914.

In this case the opinion of the Commission was divided. The local diagnosis was Yellow Fever.

The patient was a European sailor, æt. 22, on board the steamship "Ashanti." Death occurred at Burutu. He was taken ill on October 17th with fever and headache, which continued for two days, followed by a remission on the third day, when the patient felt much better. This was followed by a further rise of temperature, and death occurred on the sixth day with delirium and hyperpyrexia. On the fifth day there was profuse epistaxis. Ten grains of quinine were given three times daily on October 17th, but without effect upon the temperature.

On the 18th at 4 p.m. ten grains of bi-hydrochloride of quinine were injected intramuscularly. There was a fall of temperature on the following day, but on the 22nd it rose from 99° to 103°, 105° and 107°, when death occurred.

" *Post-mortem Examination.*

" Yellow tinge of skin: conjunctivæ tinged. Lividity of neck, trunk and back, hæmorrhage from nose. Small hæmorrhages in pericardium. Small hæmorrhagic spots in lungs.

" Mucous membrane of stomach injected with patchy swellings, no hæmorrhage into cavity. Duodenum and a patch in jejunum show congestion. Liver brownish in colour, soft, appearance of fatty degeneration. Spleen 13 oz., dark and practically diffluent and much engorged.

" Kidneys, cortex and medulla congested, R. 6 oz., L. 6 oz.

" *Post-mortem Diagnosis and Conclusions.*

" Death due to hyperpyrexia. The history of the case, length of fever with its remission on the third day and subsequent rise accompanied by nasal hæmorrhage and the light yellow staining of the skin, together with the post-mortem findings, point to the conclusion that the hyperpyrexia was due to Yellow Fever.

" 24th October, 1914."

On Board ss. "Nembe," 1914.

131. The patient was a European, æt. 14 years, a member of the crew of a steamship lying at the wharf at Burutu. The date of the onset of the illness is uncertain; death occurred from Yellow Fever on March 26th, 1914, and the diagnosis was confirmed by post-mortem examination.

The movements of the ship were as follows:—

Station.	Arrival.	Departure.	Remarks.
Sierra Leone ...	February 24th	February 24th	—
Bonny	March 3rd	March 4th	—
Port Harcourt ...	March 4th	March 11th	Alongside wharf, and in contact with ss. "Degema" from 4th–6th; and in contact with ss. "Egwanga" from 8th–11th. *Deceased was ashore.*
Calabar	March 12th	March 17th	Alongside Government wharf from 13th–17th; but not in contact with any vessels. *Deceased did not go ashore.*
Forcados	March 19th	March 22nd	In contact with ss. "Hartley" in mid-stream from 19th–22nd. No person on board went ashore.
Burutu Channel ... (stuck ashore on mud bank.)	March 22nd	March 24th	—
Burutu	March 24th	March 27th	—
Quarantine Station, Forcados ...	March 28th	—	—

No further cases occurred and no cases of a suspicious nature were reported.

The ss. "Hartley" was inspected on arrival at Lagos, but no cases of illness were found on board.

(*B*)—EPIDEMICS IN 1914.

(1) NIGERIA.—SOUTHERN PROVINCES.

(*a*) WARRI.

In Appendix D. (I.R., Vol. I., p. 307) of Dr. T. R. Russell Leonard's "Report on Certain Outbreaks of Yellow Fever in Lagos, 1913, and January and February, 1914," one case diagnosed as of Yellow Fever on board the ss. "Arnfried" at Koko, Warri, and four other cases of fever of a doubtful nature, which occurred at the same time and in the same ship are mentioned. Of these cases Dr. Leonard states:—

"From the above report Case No. 1, in my opinion, is undoubtedly a mild infection of Yellow Fever. In Cases 2 and 3, although malaria parasites were found to be present, the signs and symptoms as a whole do not present a picture of simple malarial infection, and should be regarded as distinctly suspicious. In Cases 4 and 5 there is very little doubt of their being ordinary cases of subtertian malarial fever. The reports are very meagre of details. Faget's sign is undoubtedly present in Case No. 1, and to a less extent in Cases 2 and 3, while absent in Cases 4 and 5."

(*b*) LAGOS.

Two cases of Yellow Fever occurred at Lagos in February, 1914 (*vide* I.R., Vol. I., p. 312). One patient (Case 1, Lagos L. 121) was an engineer of a vessel lying at Iddo Wharf in Lagos. The other patient was an assistant in a trading firm (Case 2, Lagos, L. 122). In August, 1913, Case No. 18 had occurred at the same factory as Case 2, and was treated in Lagos Hospital.

Lagos was put in quarantine on the occurrence of the second case.

As the Commission were divided in opinion on the first case. it may be desirable to state it in full in this Report:—

"*Name*: Mr. C.
"*Age*: 30 years.
"*Sex*: Male.
"*Nationality*: European, British.
"*Occupation*: Engineer, s.s. 'Porto Novo' from Forcados, 24th January, 1914.
"*Date of admission*: 12th February, 1914.
"*Date of discharge*: 27th February, 1914.
"*Diagnosis*: Yellow Fever.

"*History*.—Patient states that he first felt ill on the 9th February with rigors, followed by severe frontal headache and fever. There was no vomiting, but nausea was present. Patient took quinine that night and also next day, but felt no better. On the 11th, he again had rigors and a high temperature, accompanied by severe frontal headache and aching pains in the extremities. This morning he was seen by Dr. Maples, and as his temperature was 104°, he was sent to the hospital. Patient has only been out five months and this is his first tour on the Coast. He has taken quinine regularly.

"*On admission*.—Patient complained of very severe frontal headache and pains in the eyes. Conjunctivæ were red and injected. Eyes shining. Temperature was 104·2°, pulse rate 88 per minute.

" *Alimentary system.*—Tongue was furred, with clean red tip and edges. Bowels were constipated. Gums red and swollen Nausea and epigastric discomfort present, increased on pressure. Patient had no vomiting, but severe retching had been present on the day before admission. Liver and spleen were both normal in size with no tenderness on palpation.

" *Circulatory system.*—Heart sounds were normal. Pulse very slow, 88 per minute.

" *Respiratory system.*—Lungs were normal. Respirations were hurried, 36 per minute.

" *Nervous system.*—Severe frontal headache and pains in the eyes. Aching pains in the extremities. Reflexes were normal.

" *Urinary system.*—Patient stated that the urine was diminished in quantity and high coloured. On examination: Acid reaction. Sp. gr. 1010. Albumen present.

" *Blood examination.*—Few young ring forms of subtertian malaria present. *Paraplasma flavigenum* present. Differential count: Polymorphon. 72·6 per cent.; lymphocytes, 17·2 per cent.; mononuclear, 8·4 per cent.; transitionals, 1·8 per cent.

" 9 p.m. Patient passed 10 ozs. of urine, none having been passed during the day. Nausea and retching were troublesome. No vomiting. Bowels were opened after the calomel. Temperature 103·6°, pulse rate 80.

" 13th February. Patient had a restless night and only slept after a draught. Bowels were opened twice in the morning. Urine was passed, 22 ozs., and on examination was acid in reaction. Sp. gr. 1022. Albumen had increased in amount. Temperature at 8 a.m. was 100·8°, pulse 84. Nausea and epigastric discomfort still present. Scleræ are tinged with yellow. Headache and muscular pains still persist. Temperature at 8 p.m. was 99·8°, pulse rate 64.

" 14th February. Patient had a better night and feels better this morning. Nausea and epigastric discomfort still present, but much lessened. Bowels were opened. Urine passed in increased quantity. On examination: Acid in reaction. Sp. gr. 1025. Albumen present. Scleræ yellow. Temperature at 8 a.m. was 99·4°, pulse 70. At 8 p.m. it was 101·2°, pulse rate 60.

" 15th February. Patient had a restless night, temperature rose to 102·4°, pulse rate 88 per minute. At 8 a.m. temperature was 101°, pulse 84. Nausea still present. Jaundice now well marked. Urine still diminished, 33 ozs. passed in the twenty-four hours, and contains albumen. Bowels opened twice. Temperature at 8 p.m. 98·4°, pulse 72.

" 16th February. Patient had a good night. Appetite returned. Jaundice more marked. Urine is acid in reaction. Sp. gr. 1,022. No albumen present. Temperature subnormal, pulse rate 64. Bowels opened. Patient continued to progress favourably. Appetite returned. Bowels regular. Urine returned to its normal quantity. Jaundice gradually disappeared on the 21st February, and the patient was discharged cured on the 27th February."

The results of the blood examinations were as follows:—

	Feb. 12th.	13th.	15th.	16th.	17th.	18th
Parasites	Subtertian rings	Subtertian rings	0	0	0	0
Polymorphonuclears	72·6	57·4	62·2	43·2	49·8	49·2
Lymphocytes ...	17·2	26·4	25·2	30·4	31·0	30·4
Mononuclears ...	8·4	11·8	7·0	13·4	11·0	10·6
Transitionals ..	1·8	4·0	4·8	7·4	4·2	5·6
Mast. cells	—	—	0·8	0·2	—	—
Eosinophiles ...	—	0·4	—	5·4	4·0	4·2

Some blood films from this case were examined by Dr. C. M. Wenyon, Director of Research in the Tropics to the Wellcome Bureau of Scientific Research, who found them to contain subtertian malaria parasites, some of which were small and had a curiously compact structure.

The second case was classified as "Probable Yellow Fever":—

"*Name*: Mr. M.

"*Sex*: Male.

"*Age*: 27 years.

"*Nationality*: European, German.

"*Occupation*: Trader, in the employ of Messrs. W. and B.

"*Date of admission*: 14th February, 1914.

"*Date of discharge*: 27th February, 1914.

"*Diagnosis*: Yellow Fever.

"*History.*—Patient states that he felt ill yesterday, the 13th, in the morning, with chills and frontal headache. Got gradually worse during the day, and at night his temperature was 104°, with very severe headache and pains in the extremities. He was seen by his medical attendant, Dr. Maples, who gave him an intramuscular injection of quinine. He had a bad night but felt better early next morning. During the day the temperature again rose, headache became severe, nausea and epigastric discomfort was present. No vomiting until he made himself vomit to relieve the nausea. In the evening his temperature was 104°, conjunctivæ were injected and red, headache very severe and his urine on examination was albuminous. So he was sent to the hospital at 7 p.m.

"*On admission.*—Temperature was 101·8°, pulse rate 98. Conjunctivæ very injected. Complained of severe frontal headache and aching pains in the loins. Patient has only been out eight months of this, his first tour. Has taken quinine regularly.

"*Alimentary system.*—Gums red and swollen. Tongue, white dorsum, with red tip and edges. Bowels constipated. Liver and spleen both normal, no tenderness. Nausea and epigastric discomfort present. Great thirst present.

"*Circulatory system.*—Heart sounds normal. Pulse slow, 90 at 8 p.m.

"*Respiratory system.*—Lungs normal. Respirations hurried.

"*Nervous system.*—Severe frontal headache present. Aching pains in the loins. Reflexes normal.

"*Urinary system.*—Urine passed on admission. Very high coloured. Acid reaction. Sp. gr. 1030. Albumen present, high percentage. Quantity has been diminished.

"*Other systems.*—Skin sweating. Face very flushed. Conjunctivæ injected. Eyes shining. Photophobia present.

"*Blood examination.*—No malaria parasites present. *Paraplasma flavigenum* present. Differential count: Polymorphon., 61 per cent.; lymphocytes, 27·4 per cent.; mononuclear, 8·4 per cent.; transitionals, 2·8 per cent.; mast cells, ·4 per cent.

"*15th February.*—Patient had a fair night, but was restless in the early part. Bowels moved after the calomel. Urine passed but diminished in quantity, only 7 ozs. passed in the previous twenty-four hours. Highly albuminous. Temperature at 8 a.m. was 99·4°, pulse rate 88. Tube casts present in the urine. During the day, the temperature rose, and at 4 p.m. was 103·6°, pulse 100. Patient very excitable, complained of great thirst. Face very flushed and conjunctivæ were very injected. At 8 p.m. temperature was 102·4°, pulse 96.

"*16th February.*—Patient was very restless last night and only slept after a draught. Conjunctivæ very injected. Nausea troublesome. Urine still diminished and contains albumen. Patient is very nervous and complains of great thirst. Temperature at 8 a.m. was 101·6°, pulse rate 88. At 8 p.m. temperature rose to 102·8°, pulse rate 90.

"*17th February.*—Patient had a better night and slept. Is feeling much improved this morning. Temperature at 8 a.m. 100·6°, pulse 100. Headache still present, also loin pains. Urine is still diminished and contains albumen, Sp. gr. 1030, acid reaction. At 8 p.m. temperature rose to 102·4°, with pulse of 90. Thirst is lessened. Conjunctivæ still injected.

"*18th February.*—Patient had a good night and is feeling very much better. Bowels opened. Urine passed in increased quantity, and on examination still contains albumen. Conjunctival injection passing off. Scleræ are now tinged with yellow. Temperature is 99°, with pulse rate of 100.

"*19th February.*—Patient is much improved and had a good night. Temperature still 99°. Bowels opened. Urine examined and found to contain bile, but no albumen. Scleræ are now decidedly yellow. Nausea and epigastric discomfort have passed off. Appetite is returning. Urine has not yet reached the normal. Headache quite gone.

"Patient continued to gradually improve, jaundice slowly disappeared on the 24th, and patient was discharged cured on the 27th February."

Daily examinations of the blood were made until the patient was discharged, but no malarial parasites were found.

It is stated in the Notes that mosquitoes prevailed in the patient's residence, chiefly *Stegomyia.*

(11) GOLD COAST.

(*a*) SALTPOND.

Saltpond is situated on the seaboard and lies 5° 12′ N., 1° 7′ W.

Case 1.—The patient was a European, aged 30 years, the agent of a Trading Association. He was in his fourth tour of service and had been out for seven months. He had resided at Saltpond for seven weeks.

The illness commenced on 7th January, 1914, and ended fatally on 12th January.

Case 2.—On the same day, a European, aged 29 years, an agent for another trading company, was taken ill with Yellow Fever and recovered after an attack lasting five days. His bedroom was in a house 70 feet from the first case, but to windward of it. Both rooms were near a dilapidated Kroo-boy house.

Case 3.—On January 15th a European trader aged 45 years, who had been at Saltpond for seven months, was taken ill with symptoms suggestive of Yellow Fever and recovered on the fifth day. His pulse on that day was 56. This case was classified as "Possible Yellow Fever."

In a report by the Senior Sanitary Officer, the following occurs:—

> "10. Inquiries made with a view to discovering the source of infection have not so far met with any success. There does not seem to have been any unusual ill-health amongst the native population, adults or children. It may have originated from an infected person living in a very dilapidated building which lies between the German West African Trading Company and the African Association. This building is inhabited by Kroos. The suspicions would seem to be more or less justified by the fact that at no time recently had the second case ever visted the African Association building, and the presumption is that the infected mosquitoes must have come from a common source."

No further cases occurred and Saltpond was declared to be free from infection on the 2nd February, 1914.

GOLD COAST, ASHANTI.

(*b*) AYENIM.

Ayenim is a mining camp three miles from Obuasi in Ashanti and ninety-five miles from the Coast. It is described as being "in a very bad state of neglect." The native village, close by, under charge of the Government doctor, was in a satisfactory state.

Case 1.—The patient was a European, aged 44, who had completed several tours on the Coast. Until April 19th, 1914, he lived at Obuasi; on that date he removed to Ayenim. On April 25th he visited Ayenim village and again on April 29th. His illness commenced on May 4th, and death occurred on May 10th. A post-mortem examination revealed lesions typical of Yellow Fever.

The occurrence of this case led to the knowledge of other cases.

Case 2.—The patient was a European engaged at the mining camp. He accompanied Case 1 to the native village on April 25th and 29th, and was taken ill on the same day as Case 1. Recovery followed after a mild attack lasting fifteen days.

The Provincial Medical Officer and the Medical Officer of Health investigated this outbreak and reported as follows upon a death which occurred at Ayenim earlier in April, 1914:—

> "*Case* 3.—I have little doubt that H———, who died in April, was a case of Yellow Fever."—*Provincial Medical Officer.*
>
> "In my opinion the outbreak dates back to April this year. On the 12th March a European, H———, arrived out from England. He lived in Bungalow A (distant 60 yards from Bungalow B, where Case 4 occurred). He took sick on April 1st, and complained of headache and gastric trouble. Next day H——— came in to Obuasi and said that he was better. He was ill again on the following two days, but did not consider himself ill enough to send for the doctor, and did not stop work. He felt much better on the 5th (Sunday), and on the morning of the 6th went to work as usual. In the afternoon he felt much worse, and died that evening. I was told by a European that after death dark blood came from H———'s nose and mouth. I believe this to have been a case of Yellow Fever."—*Medical Officer of Health.*

The cause of death was returned by the mine doctor as "heat stroke" and he maintained that opinion. The Commission were divided in opinion as to the nature of this case; it was ultimately classified as "Negative" by a majority.

After the death of this patient, Case 1 left Obuasi, on April 19th, for Ayenim, and slept in the same room that H——— had occupied. Case 2 occupied the other room in that bungalow.

Case 4.—A European, T———, was found by the medical officers to be ill when they visited Ayenim. He lived in Bungalow B, distant 60 yards from Bungalow A.

> "He had symptoms very suspicious, in my opinion, of a mild attack of Yellow Fever, and was accordingly isolated in hospital with Case 2."—*Medical Officer of Health.*

(*c*) TAMALE.

The following are the rather scanty details of these cases:—

"CASE 1.

> "Carpenter, Public Works Department. There was much frontal headache; pain in the joints was a prominent symptom. Vomiting occurred once, on the day of admission to hospital. Epigastric tenderness was present; albumen appeared in the urine on the second day of the illness and disappeared on the following day. The urine

was very small in quantity and contained a few blood corpuscles and hyaline casts on the second day only. The pulse rate did not fall when the temperature dropped. The liver and spleen were not enlarged. The temperature on admission was 104° F., rose in the evening to 104·5° F., fell on the second day to 101° F., and became normal on the third day. No malaria parasites were found in the blood.

"CASE 2.

"Private, Northern Territories Constabulary. There was frontal headache and photophobia, very slight jaundice in the scleræ. Epigastric tenderness and a good deal of vomiting both on the first and second day of illness. Albumen was large in amount on the first day of illness, and diminished on the second and disappeared on the third day. There were a few blood corpuscles seen in the urine on the first and second days of the disease, also hyaline casts. Tongue was very furred at the back but clean at the edge. Malaria parasites were not found.

"There was no hepatic enlargements, Faget's sign was absent, but the pulse rate fell to 58, when the temperature dropped. Hyaline casts were present in the urine on both days of examination.

"The temperature on admission was 104° F., and fell to normal on the second day. Pulse 100 on admission, 58 on the second day."

Two other cases of a suspicious character but with less marked symptoms occurred about the same time.

None of these cases have been classified by the Commission.

(*C*)—OUTBREAKS IN 1915.

NIGERIA.—SOUTHERN PROVINCES.

(*a*) BURUTU.

A fatal case in a native, locally diagnosed as Yellow Fever, was reported by telegram on September 23rd, 1915.

(*b*) ONITSHA.

On September 13th, 1915, a fatal case in a native prisoner, locally diagnosed as Yellow Fever, was reported by telegram.

On September 16th a second case was reported from Onitsha, also in a native.

In consequence of these two cases Onitsha town was declared infected on September 16th. On October 9th, no fresh cases having occurred, Onitsha was declared to be free from Yellow Fever.

(*c*) ENGENNI RIVER.

On October 13th, 1915, five cases of Yellow Fever in natives were reported by telegram to have occurred at a camp known as "Engenni Concessions," on Engenni River, twenty miles from Degema.

The place was declared to be infected, and the necessary precautions were taken.

The Engenni River during the period of the year in which these cases occurred is a highway between the River Niger and Oguta, to Degema and Bonny; steamboats are then able to travel up and down the river.

The Labourers' Camp, where the two deaths took place, is situated on the right bank of the river, three miles below the village of Abumi, below its junction with the Egboribiri creek, twenty miles distant from Degema. Communication with other places is by canoe, dense forests and swamps preventing overland traffic.

None of the labourers had been away from the camp since the 16th August, 1915, with the exception of going into the uninhabited forest to fell trees; no fresh labour was imported into the camp between 16th August and 26th September.

No unusual disease was known to be prevailing at the camp before the 26th September. The history of the two fatal cases was obtained by Dr. T. R. Beale-Browne, the Medical Officer at Degema, who visited the camp immediately on the receipt, on October 8th, of information from the agent for the timber concession that two labourers had died under peculiar circumstances, and that three or four other labourers were ill.

"CASE 1.

"Akorisa.—Came to the concession as a labourer, having left Newi district at the beginning of August, and arrived on or about August 16th.

"On 25th September he was said to have been quite well, and was at work.

"On the morning of September 26th he did not look well, felt ill, and was told to rest in the camp.

"About 11 p.m. on that day he was reported to be vomiting blood and died comparatively suddenly shortly afterwards. His only complaint was of a violent headache.

"There was no history of fever, but in the report it is stated that 'all accounts are most meagre.'"

"CASE 2.

"Chukuma.—Came to the camp on the same day (August 16th) and from the same district. He was ill for three days before death. All that could be ascertained was that he was taken ill on or about the 3rd October.

"He had fever and diarrhœa and felt weak, but did not vomit. Just before death he had a convulsion. Death occurred on 5th October."

Two of the following cases were taken ill about October 6th, two about October 7th, and one on or about October 9th. All, with the exception of one, Obi (Case 6), a native of Kwali, who arrived at the Camp in January, 1915, were natives of the Onitsha district and arrived in camp on 16th August, 1915.

"CASE 3.

"*Name*: Obi Yasobili.

"*Age*: 20 (about.)

"*Occupation*: Labourer.

"*Tribe*: Ibo.

"*Previous history*: Recruited from the Onitsha district (Newi) at the beginning of August, and arrived at the timber camp about the middle of the same month, where he has been ever since.

"*History of present attack*: Became unwell on the evening of 9th October; complains of great pain in back and head; a general ache all over him.

"*Condition when seen*: A small youth of poor physique, seen on morning of 10th October; he was then suffering from severe pain in back, limbs, and head, seemed hardly able to move about. Eyes injected and puffy. Heart, lungs, spleen, and liver normal. Has passed only a little urine, and that very dark before visit; tongue narrow and red at edges but not much furred in centre. Temperature, 100·4°. Pulse, 120.

"11th October: Temperature, 103·6°. Pulse, 128; skin dry and hot, eyes still injected and yellowish. Passing only small amount of urine, the colour being very dark ('palm oil.'). This is acid in reaction—has a large amount of albumen in it and bile pigment. Has a peculiar smell.

"12th October: The symptoms are the same, violent pains, eyes are more yellow. Urine still passed, only in small amounts and very dark and albuminous.

"13th October: The peculiar smell, first noticed on 11th, is present, but not so noticeable.

"14th October: Temperature rose on this day to 101·8°; he seems no worse; urine is more freely passed.

"15th October: Temperature coming down again; urine still dark and contains albumen and bile pigment. Still has great pain in head.

"17th October: Is now much better; only a trace of albumen; says he feels all right."

"CASE 4.

"*Name*: Peter.
"*Age*: 23 (about).
"*Occupation*: Labourer.
"*Tribe*: Ibo.

"*Previous history*: Recruited at beginning of August in the Onitsha district and arrived in the timber camp about middle of same month, where he has resided ever since.

"*History of present attack*: Had pain in head and legs, also knees, about 7th October, the exact date is a little uncertain. The interpretation was very poor and much trouble in getting details.

"*Condition when seen*: Says he is better, but has a headache and pains in knees and lower parts of legs. The heart, lungs, spleen, and liver normal. Temperature, 100·4°. Pulse, 102. Eyes seemed normal, slight injection. On 10th October scleræ were yellowish. Urine was pale and clear—alkaline, trace of albumen.

"12th October: Seems to be quite well and feeling well. Complaining as he did, and seeing condition of his fellow sick, he was classed as Yellow Fever, but if seen by himself he would not have been so diagnosed."

"CASE 5.

"*Name*: Obashuru.
"*Age*: 22 (about).
"*Occupation*: Labourer.
"*Tribe*: Ibo.

"*Previous history*: Was recruited in the Onitsha district—near Newi—in the beginning of August, 1915. He arrived at the timber camp on or about 16th August. He gives no account of previous fever similar to what he is now suffering from.

"*History of present attack*: On or about 6th October he complained of pain in the back and legs and felt ill. He had fever. Bowels were not acting well, so had a dose of salts which acted well.

"*Condition when seen*: A poor, weak specimen. Complains of great aching pain in back and limbs, especially legs. His eyes are congested with a yellow tinge.

"Tongue is very narrow, rather dry—red at edges and the centre furred. Heart, lungs, liver appear normal. Spleen is a little enlarged. Urine, which was small in amount, is now being passed better. It is of a dark brown colour, like 'palm oil'; the froth is yellow. Reaction acid, albumen was present in large quantity. Bile pigment, also on 10th; the day after first seen his eyes were much yellower.

"This state of affairs continued—only the urine increased in quantity and less dark in colour till 16th October, when urine was normal. He was then feeling well but weak. Eyes still yellow, but fading.

"The symptoms that he most complained of were persistent headache. There was no vomiting: Faget's sign was not present."

"Case 6.

"*Name*: Obi.
"*Age*: 23 (about).
"*Occupation*: Labourer.
"*Tribe*: Ibo.

"*Previous history*: He came from the Kwali district in about January, 1915, and came to the timber camp, where he has been ever since, his work being to go into the forest to cut timber. He had no communication with the local natives, as the camp is isolated. Says he has never had, or seen people with an illness like what he has had.

"*History of present attack*: On or about 6th October, 1915, he became ill with severe pains in stomach, back, and head, but says he has not had fever (interpretation is bad).

"*Condition when seen*: Complains of great pain in stomach, chest, back and head. Tongue is red, but not the peculiar narrow red edged. Spleen normal. Heart, lungs, liver, normal; eyes are yellow and somewhat injected. The urine was small in amount, very dark, colour of 'palm oil'; loaded with albumen, and with bile pigment.

"12th October: The specific gravity of urine was 1015 (urinometer is questionable); acid, still dark, and containing albumen and bile, but only in small amount compared to previous samples. The symptom most complained of was frontal headache, otherwise he said he felt well.

"13th October: Said he felt all right, only a trace of albumen in the urine. Eyes have only a yellow tinge.

"15th October: No albumen in urine, says he feels all right."

"Case 7.

"*Name*: Obioko.
"*Age*: 22 (about).
"*Occupation*: Labourer.
"*Tribe*: Ibo.

"*Previous history*: Recruited in the Onitsha district (Newi) at beginning of August, and arrived in timber camp about 16th August, 1915. He has had no communication with the local inhabitants.

"*History of present attack*: Has been unwell since 6th or 7th October, with great pains in epigastric area and back. There is no history of vomiting. Has had a cough recently.

"*Condition when seen 9th October*: Complains of great pain in stomach and back and head. Conjunctivæ puffy and injected. Tongue narrow, bright red at edges, furred in centre. Heart, normal. Lungs, some râles and rhonchi. Spleen, slight enlargement; liver normal. Urine very dark ('palm oil'), acid; large amount of albumen and bile pigment.

"10th October: Lungs clear; urine the same, also symptoms. Temperature, 101·8°. Pulse, 95. Eyes yellowish.

"12th October: Eyes still injected but more yellow; albumen in the urine, also bile.

"13th October: Urine pale, acid; trace of albumen.

"15th October: Urine to-day was much darker and had a greenish yellow tinge; trace of albumen and bile pigment.

"18th October: Is now all right; feeling well, only a little weak."

The following extracts are from the Report of Dr. T. R. Beale-Browne, Medical Officer at Degema, to the Principal Medical Officer, Lagos. It is possible that owing to the prompt action taken the outbreak was prevented from developing into a serious epidemic, but before accepting it as proved that this was the case it would be necessary to know whether the labourers not affected had, by previous attacks, been rendered immune to the disease.

"PRECAUTIONARY MEASURES TAKEN.

"1. Immediately it was appreciated that the illness was not an ordinary one, the huts were as efficiently stopped up as possible and sulphur candles burnt.

"Certain huts were apportioned to the sick, with orders that they lived by themselves, all the other labourers to keep apart.

"The sick were kept under mosquito nets; the difficulties of taking these apparently simple precautions were great. Rain pouring all day—for days—the camp being more or less under water. The only way to get about the camp was wading in inches of mud and water. The huts were of a very poor construction; added to this, the river was rising. This caused great trouble in the new camp formed three miles lower down the river.

"2. As the floors that were to be were under water quite soon, this necessitated raising the inside of the houses.

"3. As soon as the labourers who were well had made sufficient shelters to protect them from the rain in the new camp they all left. Then the huts they had occupied were burnt down.

"4. Leaving only the contractor's house, which the sick then occupied.

"5. In addition to these local precautions, more general ones were taken. The District Officer, Ahoada, arranged for traffic from his district not to go to the infected area; a patrol being set to stop canoes going down or up.

"6. At the Degema end all traffic was held up from down the Engenni as much as possible, but, for determined people, it was easy to evade the guard, as there are so many creeks; so the District Officer, Degema, called a meeting of all the Abonnema chiefs, and, with the Medical Officer, the whole matter was put before them, and the whole of Abonnema was divided up so as to have the whole place watched, and all canoes coming from Oguta way to either go back or land and be quarantined.

"All natives on their farms on the river were told that they must not go to the infected camp.

"There were very few people on these river farms as the water was so high."

* * * * *

"7. Insects.—In the old camp, mosquitoes were breeding everywhere. All the larvæ at first collected were *Culex* and *Anopheles*, and only a few of the latter. As time went on, and the ground began to dry, in the few places that escaped being paraffined, with few exceptions, the larvæ hatched out into *Anophelines*.

"Endeavours to find *Stegomyia* were fruitless; the mat roofing was disturbed and an entomological net waved to catch anything, but no mosquito was caught. Many of the ponds or puddles were treated with kerosene, but this was limited.

"The bush around was beaten and all flying things caught, but this was resultless as far as mosquitoes. Nevertheless as soon as evening approached the whole place swarmed with mosquitoes and sand-flies. Personally I only saw *Anophelines*, and I also always left the camp before sunset.

"Of other biting flies *Tabanidæ* are very common, and only a very few tsetse flies have been seen, and the latter near Degema."

The following extract is from the Report of the Principal Medical Officer to the Secretary, Southern Provinces, Lagos:—

"9. There is no evidence of the introduction of the disease from without.

"10. No further cases have occurred.

"11. In my opinion, these cases add further proof of the occurrence of Yellow Fever among the natives of Nigeria. Indeed, there can be no question of their immunity, the evidence of their susceptibility is steadily increasing, though they may have it in a remarkably mild form."

These cases have not been classified by the Commission.

The following case, which occurred in January, 1914, is inserted here, as it acquires additional interest from the outbreak of Yellow Fever reported above.

It will be seen that whereas the pathological report states that there was evidence of advanced alcoholic cirrhosis of the liver, a complication of the most dangerous character in **any** case of Yellow Fever, yet the substance of the organ is stated in the post-mortem report to have been "soft and friable and flabby in the extreme." These conditions are hardly consistent with advanced alcoholic cirrhosis. It must, however, be remembered that decomposition may proceed very rapidly after death in the tropics.

The deceased was employed on the Engenni River, and had gone up the river from Degema.

"REPORT OF A CASE FROM DR. TIPPER, ONITSHA.

., Vol. I., 311-312. "The body of a European was brought into Onitsha at 11.30 p.m. on the 13th January, 1914, death having occurred shortly before, outside Onitsha, at Newi. A letter that accompanied the deceased stated that he had been suffering from 'bilious fever' for some days previously, and had been treated by the Medical Officer at Ogouta, and that quinine had been used.

"Autopsy was performed 16 hours after death.

"*Skin.*—Universally bright yellow in colour. Conjunctivæ showing hæmorrhagic injection at lower and outer corneo-sclerotic junction. Seleræ bright yellow. Undue post-mortem staining of the right arm and dependent parts of the back and legs. There was some dark red blood streaming from the angle of the mouth which had obviously been vomited.

"*Stomach.*—A bluish-black, semi-coagulated mucus covered the surface of the interior. Here and there was seen very dark coloured blood, similar to that found issuing from the mouth. The mucous membrane was of a black colour but mottled, the black portions alternating with the red patches. The rugæ were easily broken. The peritoneal surface was almost black, but dull red patches and ecchymoses occurred here and there.

"*Liver.*—A bright yellow ochre colour. The anterior parts of the under surfaces of the right and left lobes were black. On section, bright yellow. The substance of the organ was soft and friable and flabby in the extreme.

"*Lungs.*—These were universally black, soft and friable. On the lower lobe of the left lung there was a large patch of blood extravasation into the pleura. No pneumonic or other consolidation present. Sections floated in water.

"*Intestines.*—Dirty yellowish white in colour. Peritoneal surface showed subperitoneal hæmorrhages. Mucous membrane had a bruised appearance due to the blood within the interstices of the tissues.

"*Heart.*—The whole organ was flabby, fat was bright yellow in colour. Muscular fibres were deep red in colour. Valves were normal.

"*Spleen.*—Slightly enlarged, softer than normal.

"*Kidneys.*—Slightly enlarged, pale yellowish infiltration of the cortex.

"*Bladder.*—Empty, normal.

"*Brain.*—Congested, ventricles contained fluid of a light lemon colour.

"LABORATORY REPORT.

"*Spleen.*—Congested, some black pigment present.

"*Brain.*—Congested, round-celled infiltration present.

"*Liver.*—Advanced necrotic changes, fatty degeneration present.

"*Kidney.*—Epithelium of convoluted tubules necrosed and desquamated in parts; elsewhere showing cloudy swelling and marked fatty changes. Glomerular tufts swollen and congested. Lumen of tubules mostly blocked by desquamated cells and debris.

"*Previous history of the case.*—The deceased was employed on a survey of the Engenni River and had gone up the river from Degema. He left the vessel at Akara Queri on the 2nd January, and proceeded to Ogouta, where he arrived on the 6th. He got ill at Ogouta, and suffered from fever with vomiting. On the 9th he was seen by the Medical Officer, Owerri, who apparently formed the opinion that he was suffering from 'bilious remittent fever.' The Medical Officer was called away on the 10th, and on the 13th the patient seemed to have become delirious and was sent off in a hammock by the Agent at Ogouta to Onitsha Hospital, but patient died shortly before arriving there.

"The infection in this case was contracted at some point between Degema and Ogouta, possibly on the ship itself or at some native town where the deceased had stayed on the way up to Ogouta. No blood examination records, or any notes or temperature chart of the case are available."

NOTE BY COMMISSION.

"Pathological material from this case was examined by Dr. A. C. Stevenson, of the Wellcome Bureau of Scientific Research, who made the following report:—

"*Liver.*—Fairly advanced cirrhosis—lobules practically indistinguishable—areas of fatty degeneration. Other areas, larger, show well-marked necrosis, some, no doubt, due to post-mortem change. No signs of acidophilic change. Pigment, malarial in appearance; soluble in acid alcohol.

"*Kidney*.—Advanced cirrhotic change; thickened capsule with fibrous tissue spreading from it between the tubules. Marked thickening of Bowman's capsule. Cloudy swelling of convoluted tubules towards the surface of the kidney. Straight tubules full of desquamated epithelial cells. In some parts of intermediate zone complete necrosis (? partly post-mortem). Desquamation in tubules of papillary region. Concretions in some tubules. Pigment, malarial in appearance, in Malpighian tufts; soluble in acid alcohol.

"*Spleen*.—Congested, excess of small round cells. Some fibrous increase and thickening of vessel walls. Malaria-like pigment.

"*Brain*.—? softening—many round spaces in some of which are bacteria which are also seen in blood vessels (? post-mortem). A fair number of concretions (psammomata). Capillaries mostly empty—small vessels engorged. In the endothelial cells of the capillaries small quantities of malaria-like pigment are seen.

"REMARKS.—No definite signs of Yellow Fever, but those of advanced alcoholism."

(*D*)—ANALYSIS OF EPIDEMICS.

(1) INCIDENCE ON EUROPEANS AND NATIVES.

We have analysed the various epidemics with which we are now concerned in order to illustrate the incidence of the disease, so far as the information is available, upon Europeans and natives. Two very important facts have, however, to be borne in mind in order to avoid erroneous conclusions from these data, viz.:—

(1) The probability of a case of Yellow Fever being recognised as such is infinitely greater in a European than in a native, and

(2) The European population in most of the large towns is, from a numerical point of view, almost negligible as compared with the native.

The greater case mortality in the Lagos epidemic of 1913 amongst the Europeans as compared with the natives is very striking, but only confirms what has been so often observed elsewhere.

That it does not obtain to anything like the same degree in the other epidemics is presumptive evidence that not nearly all the native cases were recognised:—

1910.

Sierra Leone, Freetown:—	Cases.	Deaths.
Syrians	9	9
Europeans	7	5
Natives	4	2
Gold Coast, Seccondee:—		
Europeans	10	9
Natives	2	2
Hausa	1	1
Saw mills:—		
European	1	
Axim:—		
European	1	
Nigeria, Lagos:—		
Natives	2	

1911.

Gold Coast, Accra:—	Cases.	Deaths.
Europeans	7	7
Natives	3	0
Avrebroo:—		
European	1	
Gambia, Bathurst:—		
Europeans	12	10
Syrians	3	2

1912.

Gold Coast, Accra:—	Cases.	Deaths.
European	3	2
Native	1	1
Zabadie:—		
European	1	
Seccondee:—		
European	1	
Axim:—		
Native	1	

1913.

Nigeria, Lagos:—	Cases.	Deaths.
Europeans	15	7
Natives	20	0
Syrians	3	2

1914.

Lagos:—	Cases.	Deaths.
Europeans	2	0
Natives	0	0

(II.) INCIDENCE ON COAST TOWNS AND TOWNS OF THE INTERIOR.

Although it is true that all the epidemics of 1910-1911, 1912 and 1913 occurred in towns on the coast that fact is not necessarily of great significance, as with the exception of Coomassie nearly all the large towns in the West African Dependencies* are situated upon the coast, and it is only in a large town, and one in which there are a certain number of Europeans, that the occurrence of an epidemic is likely to attract attention.

In the Second Report (p. 135) under the heading "Epidemics of Yellow Fever of a severe type amongst natives" the following occurs:—

> "At the same time other and at first sight contradictory evidence is increasing, tending to show that amongst the natives living in regions either distant from the coast, or from the European settlements on the coast, epidemics of a disease which cannot be distinguished from Yellow Fever are of occasional occurrence, and that such epidemics are attended with a very high mortality."

Four examples of these are given, and they still remain the only outbreaks of the kind of which we are aware.

If these epidemics were really due to Yellow Fever, and no other disease capable of producing such a clinical picture is known, it would appear to be possible that the natives of Africa living in the interior possess a lesser degree of insusceptibility to the disease than those of the coast.

It is by no means improbable that this should be so, as the disease has, so long as we know something of its history, always prevailed upon the coast, and, speaking generally, any people which has been for many generations attacked at frequent intervals by an epidemic disease is likely to possess a higher degree of resistance to it than one not so circumstanced.

The large number of sporadic outbreaks which have been reported since the appointment of the Commission is, however, as already stated, clear proof of the wide distribution of the disease during that period, and it is extremely unlikely that they represent anything exceptional, save a wider recognition of the endemic presence of the disease.

---

* Only one case is known to have occurred in the Northern Province of Nigeria.

(III.) INCIDENCE ON NEW-COMERS, EUROPEAN AND AFRICAN.

(*a*) From Outside Africa.

Yellow Fever is pre-eminently a disease affecting new-comers.

The first case in the Freetown epidemic of 1910 was a Syrian, and seven deaths occurred amongst Syrians between April 17th and May 25th. These were not all classified as "Yellow Fever" for reasons already given (*vide* p. 47), but there can be little doubt that they were all fatal from that disease.

In the commentary upon this epidemic (Second Report, p. 113) the following appears:—

> "(1) A knowledge of the movements of the Syrian (Case 1) for (say) six weeks prior to April 17th would be of interest, but there is no reason to believe that he landed from an infected ship. There is no evidence that the disease was imported. Six fatal cases had occurred amongst the Syrians before an Englishman was attacked; he had been 'long resident in Freetown.'
>
> "Europeans and Syrians, naturally, in West Africa constitute almost entirely the 'New-comer' class, but this is not tantamount to stating that they are all recent arrivals, as some of them may have been on the coast, with intervals of absence, for many years."

Several instances are mentioned in the course of this Report of two cases occurring about the same time and at the same place, one fatal, the other ending in recovery, in which the patient who died was a recent arrival, and the patient who recovered had been some time on the Coast.

(*b*) From the Hinterland to the Coast.

Freetown Epidemic, 1910.

One of the Syrians (Case 8) amongst whom this epidemic began had been travelling in the Protectorate before the onset of his illness, and may be considered as at the time a newcomer to the Coast.

Case 11, a Government official, was a new-comer in two aspects—firstly, as being without tropical experience, having only been six and a half months on the Coast, and, secondly, as having recently been travelling in the Protectorate. He was taken ill at Yonni in the Moyamba district, and is classed as an "ambulant" case.

In the Seccondee epidemic of 1910 Cases 28 and 29 were natives, but not resident in Seccondee.

At Accra in 1911, Cases 43 and 44 were non-native of Accra, but both patients had been in Accra for some months.

(*c*) FROM OTHER PARTS OF THE COAST.

In the Seccondee epidemic of 1910 it is possible that the disease was introduced from Accra.

In the same year the disease was probably carried from Seccondee to Axim, but no further case occurred there. In the same year after the outbreak at Seccondee was at an end, a patient who died from Yellow Fever was brought to that town from Saw Mills Camp, 12½ miles by rail, but there was no recrudescence of the disease at Seccondee.

In 1910 the disease was brought to Lagos from Ilesha by a native who died. Nine days later another negro died from the same cause at Lagos. Both these cases were classified as "Probably Yellow Fever."

In 1912 the disease was probably carried from Accra to Weshiang, but no further cases occurred.

(IV.) INCIDENCE ON SAILORS AND PEOPLE HAVING TO DO WITH SHIPPING.

In the outbreak at Warri in 1913 both the patients were employed on shore, and slept in their own quarters, but as they were agents of trading firms and worked in a store close to the beach, they are included in the class of people who have to do with shipping.

No light was thrown upon the source of infection in these cases, and neither of the patients had been absent from Warri for more than a month before the onset of the illness. There was no suspicion of the disease having been introduced by an infected ship, but in discussing these cases it is noted that "the facilities for conveyance of *Stegomyia* to the premises of the firm in question by water transport are considerable."

„ Vol. I., 156-177. In Section III. of Dr. E. J. Wyler's 4th Report the nature of 33 cases of fever on ocean-going vessels and dredgers in 1912 and 1913 is discussed at length. Six of these were natives of West Africa, the others were Europeans, all except one being sailors. Twelve of these cases were diagnosed locally as Yellow Fever, the remaining twenty-one were not so diagnosed, but of them it is stated that whilst "some are characterised merely by certain suggestive features, others are undoubtedly highly suspicious."

(v.) EFFECT OF TRAFFIC BY LAND AND BY SEA AND CHANGES THAT HAVE TAKEN PLACE IN THE COURSE OF YEARS.

The introduction of railways has no doubt increased the possibilities of transference of the disease from an infected area to places distant and either at the time, and possibly hitherto, free from infection. The Abeokuta case (*vide* p. 54) was closely investigated from this point of view, and it appeared that the average number of natives travelling per day between that place and Iddo (the railway terminus for Lagos) during March, April and May, 1913, was 110. The journey occupies between three and four hours. It did not, however, appear that any suspicious cases or suspicious high mortality had occurred on the line of railway between those two places.

Dr. Wyler discusses the possibility of the disease having been introduced into Abeokuta viâ the Dahomey-Nigeria boundary, and shows that in the villages and towns which would most naturally be selected by a trader as stopping places *Stegomyia fasciata* are to be found.

The traffic between Dahomey and Abeokuta is constant, and the routes are various. If therefore Dahomey should prove to be an endemic area (*vide* p. 244) the occurrence of cases in Abeokuta ceases to be as astonishing as at the time it seemed.

(vi.) EFFECT OF THE SEASON OF THE YEAR.

The exceptional prevalence in West Africa of severe types of fever, variously named, at the time of "the rains" has long been observed. The following references to this fact occur in Dr. Lind's work, and are quoted in the Second Report (p. 17):—

> "I am informed by a surgeon who practised some years at Senegal that for several months of the year during the dry season the country was as healthy and pleasant as any in the world: but soon after the rainy season began a low malignant fever constantly spread itself among the Europeans."

"The most mortal epidemic, however, is that low malignant fever of the remitting kind which rages only in the rainy season."

The despatch of the Governor of Sierra Leone, quoted on p. 32 of the Second Report, begins as follows:—

"During the months of May and June the season of heavy rains sets in on this portion of the African Coast, after an almost uninterrupted period of drought of about five months' duration. Experience has shown that during the early period of this rainy season the malarious influences of the soil, which are at all times powerful, show a marked increase in activity and virulence. Cases of malarious fever become more than usually numerous, and the disease itself, in many instances, assumes a more than ordinarily severe form. The history of Sierra Leone shows that, at intervals, seasons have recurred which have been marked by exceptional unhealthiness and by the development of the ordinary malarious fever into fevers of a most malignant type."

It would seem, however, from what appears in a medical report enclosed in the same despatch that, at any rate, as regards Yellow Fever, this dependence upon the rains was not invariable, *e.g.*, "In 1823 Yellow Fever was epidemic, commencing in the earlier part of the year, the so-called healthy or 'dry season,' and running on through the early rains and ending with the 'heavy rains.'"

The epidemic of 1829 was stated to have been "most prevalent during the blowing of the westerly winds and the falling of the heavy rain."

In 1837 the disease "commenced amongst the Europeans in the month of April, but many very suspicious cases of endemic, remittent, and the so-called African fever, occurred during the month of January, and two cases died having distinct black vomit."

The following extracts are from Staff-Surgeon Gore's Report (*vide* p. 31):—

"The first case amongst the troops was on May 11th (1837). The violence of the disease declined with the maturity of the rains. The interval between the occurrence of new cases gradually decreased with the saturation of the ground and atmosphere with moisture, until it quietly ceased * * * * * *."

"In 1847 the disease appeared epidemically in Freetown during June, July and August: only 38·85 ins. of rain had fallen in these months, and hot dry days were of frequent occurrence."

"In 1866 when the heavy rains set in they succeeded in arresting the spread of the malignant fever, which during the early weeks of the quarter ending June 30th was so fatal to the inhabitants."

The following paragraph summarises and repeats the conclusions:—

> "While the rainy season (June, July, August, September) must be considered the most unhealthy and that during which, as a rule, the ordinary fevers are most prevalent and severe, particularly at its commencement and close, it is equally certain that when the rains are slight and intermittent, grave forms of disease frequently occur, more especially of the Malignant, Remittent or Paludal Yellow Fever. This disease has almost always been arrested by a heavy rainfall in Freetown. Isolated cases have been observed during the rains, but very rarely. The heavy rain usually causes it to merge into the ordinary remittents of the Colony, in some years exhausting itself in these forms; in others only lying dormant and again appearing at the close of the wet season. The ships belonging to the naval squadron, isolated timber and other vessels have been occasionally visited by extraordinary outbreaks of remittent fever, although distinct from the malignant Yellow Fever which has at times prevailed epidemically in this Colony, have nevertheless occasionally almost rivalled that disease in its great characteristic of deadliness. They have always occurred at the close of the rainy season or immediately after."

It is probable that "an extraordinary outbreak of fever characterised by great deadliness" occurring in those days at Sierra Leone was really Yellow Fever.

In 1894, at Freetown, malarial fever of a pernicious type appeared in February, and prevailed in May, June, July and August.

There are numerous records of the prevalence of Yellow Fever at Freetown and elsewhere on the coast during these latter months.

In Senegambia there are records of the occurrence of Yellow Fever "in the early part of the year" in 1900 and 1911, and cases continued to occur in January, February and March, 1912.

In the Soudan the epidemic of 1828 is said to have begun at Christmas. On the Ivory Coast there was an epidemic in 1857 which began in February, and in 1903 another which commenced in January.

In 1896 an epidemic of a malignant type of fever was prevalent during the first four months of the year on the Gold Coast.

In 1905 in Togoland, cases of Yellow Fever occurred in January and February, and in the same year, and during the same months, at Agoué, Ouidah and Grand Popo in Dahomey.

Assistant Surgeon Eames (*vide* Second Report, page 89) records an outbreak on the River Bonny in March, 1862, which was fatal to 130 white inhabitants out of 163 in three months.

The above evidence, which might easily be increased, is sufficient to prove that in the past Yellow Fever has not been limited to the period of "the rains," although it is certainly more prevalent at that period of the year.

The following table shows the months in which the epidemics of 1910 and the succeeding years began and ended:—

	Began.	Ended.
	1910.	
Freetown ...	April 7th ...	September 15th.
Gold Coast ...	March 10th ...	May 25th.
Axim	July 6th	—
Sawmills ...	July 18th	—
Lagos	July 26th ...	August 5th.
	1911.	
Accra	February 19th ...	June 22nd.
Avreboo ...	June 22th ...	—
Gambia ...	May 18th ...	November 21st.
	1912.	
Accra ...	April 10th ...	June 27th.
Labadi ...	July 19th	—
Seccondee ...	May 17th	—
Axim	December 5th ...	—
	1913.	
Grand Popo ...	February 19th ...	March 12th.
Accra .	March 15th ...	April 14th.
Warri	June 13th ...	June 30th.
Accra	June 16th ...	July 3rd.
Lagos ...	July 21st ...	September 16th.
Lagos ...	October 4th ...	November 5th.

For all the above periods quarantine was declared.

The following are single cases for which quarantine was not declared:—

	1913.
Saltpond	January 18th
Grand Popo—Agoué (Dahomey) ...	May 2nd
Abokobi (Gold Coast)	May 14th
Quittah (Gold Coast)	July 2nd
Lome (Togoland)	September 13th
Foreados (Southern Nigeria)	October 20th
Lagos	November 26th
,, ...	December 24th
,, ...	December 28th

It would appear therefore that although by far the greater number of epidemics of Yellow Fever on the West Coast of Africa have occurred during the rainy season, yet there is no month in the year during which the disease may not be met with, even in an epidemic form.

If we assume the correctness of these various observations, and there appears to be no reason for not doing so, as they are confirmed by experience on other parts of the West African coast and elsewhere, they can be explained in the light of our present day knowledge of the two diseases, Malaria and Yellow Fever, with which we are certainly and mainly dealing, by the fact that speaking generally the conditions described favour the multiplication of mosquitoes, both *Anophelines* and *Stegomyia*, and therefore tend to favour the incidence of the diseases of which they are the carriers. It is not, however, at first sight so easy to explain the statement that slight and intermittent rains favour the occurrence of epidemics of Yellow Fever.

Some researches of Mr. Bacot, which are described in the section on Mosquitoes (*vide* p. 220), throw a new light upon the influence of moisture and rainfall in producing a sudden increase in the number of mosquitoes, and afford a probable explanation of the connection between a slight rainfall and disease on the West Coast of Africa.

The researches of Mr. Malcolm Evan MacGregor at the Wellcome Research Bureau on the life history of *Stegomyia* bred from the eggs on the dried leaves sent home by Mr. Bacot, are also of great interest (*vide* p. 235).

(VII.) INTERVALS BETWEEN EPIDEMICS.

"The History of Yellow Fever," by Augustin, to which frequent reference is made in the Second Report, contains a summary of the Yellow Fever years, and the periods of immunity in Africa from 1494 to 1907.

It cannot be supposed for a moment that the list of epidemics therein given really represents the true incidence of the disease on that part of the world during that period, but it is probable that few severe epidemics amongst Europeans in the later years have been omitted. What was happening amongst the natives at the same time is unfortunately not known.

Starting at the year 1778, which for reasons given in the Historical Retrospect (*vide* Second Report) we have fixed as the earliest trustworthy record of its presence on the Coast, we find that in the 130 following years 70 Yellow Fever years are included.

The number of these years contained in each decade is as follows:—

	Epidemic years.
1778-1787	3
1788-1797	1
1798-1807	3
1808-1817	6
1818-1827	9
1828-1837	4
1838-1847	5
1848-1857	7
1858-1867	8
1868-1877	4
1878-1887	6
1888-1897	4
1898-1907	10
130	70

During the following periods, viz.:—

From 1821 to 1830
" 1852 " 1860
" 1862 " 1869
" 1897 " 1907

the disease was continuously in evidence.

In the table showing the incidence of Yellow Fever in the West African Dependencies from 1900 to 1914 given in the Second Report (*vide* page 139) the only year in which it seems to have been absent is 1909, the year immediately preceding the epidemics which attracted special attention, and led to the appointment of the Commission.

During the period from 1778 to 1907 the longest interval of apparent freedom was from 1793 to 1803, eleven years; the next was from 1831 to 1836, six years; the total of the free years is 60.

A study of the periods of prevalence and of apparent freedom gives no indication of the existence of any cycle or law of periodical recurrence, and it is very unlikely that such exists.

---

* Evidence has since been obtained of the presence of the disease at Phillipville, in French Gaboon, in July, 1909.

It is, however, highly significant that from 1897 to 1914, a period during which attention has been much directed to tropical diseases, Yellow Fever has been continuously observed in the Dependencies on the West African coast, with the exception of only one year.*

In the Second Report (page 37), under Sierra Leone, a list is given of the periods between the years 1807 and 1884 during which no mention is made, in a report of the latter date, of the presence of Yellow Fever in that Colony. The intervals vary in duration from four to ten years, and it is remarked that "it would be of great interest to determine whether the disease was really absent during these periods, but it is very unlikely that the most diligent search amongst the records would bring to light evidence of a convincing character." It is the same with every other Dependency upon the West Coast.

The Commission has elicited no evidence which either proves or suggests that during these intervals the disease is continuously present either amongst the Europeans or amongst the native inhabitants of every place where its presence, at some time or other, has been recognised. It may be there, but the fact has not been *proved*, and it is, in their opinion, more probable that continuity is maintained by the existence of endemic areas and endemic foci than by its continuous and universal prevalence in a mild form amongst the native population, in the same way that Malaria may be said to be continuously and almost universally present.

Such foci may also conceivably lead, through movements of man or mosquito, to the establishment of new or secondary foci, in which a similar "smouldering" of infection may be maintained.

The fact, which has been proved, over and over again, during the period covered by the work of the Commission, that the natives, as a whole, are susceptible to Yellow Fever, although they usually have it in a mild form, is conclusive against the theory of its universal prevalence amongst them. Having regard to the rarity of second attacks occurring in the same individual, it is clear that Yellow Fever belongs to that class of diseases which is characterised by the fact that, as a rule, immunity is conferred by a single attack. Exceptions occur, however, in the case of each of these diseases; and there is no reason to believe that the exceptions are more numerous in the case of Yellow Fever than with the others; indeed,

* But *vide* footnote on opposite page.

it is probably true that they are less numerous. No onc, indeed, denies that in the separate towns of each Colony, in which Yellow Fever has at some time appeared, there are periods during which it is not present among the Europeans. It is not, however, so easy to disprove its continued presence amongst the natives.

The question of real interest is, "What happens to the virus in these intervals of absence or inactivity?"

Upon this it is easy to speculate and advance theories, but so long as we lack the means of identifying with certainty the minor manifestations of the disease amongst the natives, all such labour is useless.

It may, however, be well to point out that we know just as little of the life history of the virus of such a common affection as Measles, although the opportunities of observing and studying that disease have been immeasurably greater than with Yellow Fever. Measles appears in, say, a village, the epidemic runs its course and the disease disappears from the village, but not from the country. After an interval of varying duration it reappears, without in many cases the source of reinfection being discovered, yet it is not suggested that it has really been present in the village all the time.*

But in a country in which a disease is constantly met with, the virus, if not again and again introduced, must in some way be kept in a condition of potential activity.

Apart from some animal, or man or the mosquito, and the native must be the man, and the *Stegomyia* the mosquito, we have no knowledge as to how this can be effected in such a disease as Yellow Fever, and naturally it is around man and the mosquito, both known to be concerned, that discussion centres as the possible "reservoir."

How the solution of this difficult problem may possibly be reached is discussed in the section of the report dealing with "Suggestions for further research" (*vide* page 253).

SECTION VIII.

TYPES OF THE DISEASE IN THE WEST AFRICAN DEPENDENCIES.

In the Second Report (p. 129) we have already discussed the clinical types of Yellow Fever as observed in various parts of the world.

---

* We hear, however, that the suggestion is about to be made.

The concluding paragraphs of that section are as follows:—

"From Ocean Springs as a centre Yellow Fever was carried to nine states and forty-two cities. The total number of cases officially recorded from September 4th, 1897, to December 25th, 1897, was 4,426, and the deaths numbered 494. In these figures the cases variously given as 500, 600 and 700, which occurred before the disease was officially recognised, are not included.

"It would be difficult to find a more complete illustration than is afforded by the record of this epidemic of the occurrence in a negroid population of Yellow Fever as a mild disease, and of the dire events which may follow failure to recognise its earliest appearance, even though it should present itself in that seemingly innocent garb. This mild form occurs in West Africa, where hitherto only the appearance in Europeans of the type accompanied by hæmorrhage has been considered sufficient to justify a diagnosis of 'Yellow Fever.'"

(*A*) MILD TYPE IN NATIVES.

Having regard to the great difficulty attending the diagnosis of the disease in cases of the mild type occurring in natives, it is fortunate that we are able to give the details of four cases of the kind which have been brought to the notice of the Commission, and which are not open to question.

Case 1.—A man with a normal temperature, and whose blood was free from malarial parasites, was injected with 1 cc. of blood from a patient with Yellow Fever in the second day of the disease. Two days later the volunteer had rigors and pyrexia; two days later he complained of headache and backache, and albumen appeared in the urine. Jaundice appeared on the fifth day. In from six to seven days all these symptoms passed off.

Case 2.—Blood from Case 1 taken on the second day of his illness, was injected intramuscularly into a second volunteer, and similar symptoms appeared and disappeared.

Case 3.—Blood from Case 2, taken on the second day of his illness, was injected into a third volunteer, and similar symptoms appeared and disappeared.

Case 4.—A similar proceeding, taking the blood of Case 3, resulted in a very mild attack. The albuminuria lasted only two days.

Case 5.—Blood from Case 4, injected into the fifth patient, produced no reaction whatever

It had been suggested that the virulence of the infection in Yellow Fever increased with its passage through ***non-immunes*** and diminished in its passage through natives. These cases, so far as they go, lend support to that theory. It is, of course, possible that the absence of any reaction in Case 5 may have been due to the fact that the patient was completely immune.

These natives are reported to have stated that they knew this fever, which was "big fever" in children, but "small" in adults, "white man would die of it, but they would not."

The following case, classified as "Probable Yellow Fever," is of this type:—

Vol. I., "CASE NO. 3. L. 25.

24–227. "*Sex*: Male.

"*Age*: 29 years.

"*Nationality*: Negro, Effik tribe.

"*Occupation*: Labourer.

"*Date of admission*: 15th May, 1913.

"*Date of discharge*: 30th May.

"*Diagnosis*: Mild yellow fever.

"*History.*—Patient, a labourer working at the Customs, came to the out-patient department at 12 noon on the 15th May, complaining of severe frontal headache and pyrexia. His temperature was 102° and he seemed greatly distressed. He stated that he had been ill for the past six days, and unable to go to his work.

"*On admission.*—Patient was in great distress, respirations hurried. Sweating freely. Conjunctivæ injected. Temperature 102°, pulse rate 98. Complains of severe headache and aching pains in the loins and all over the body.

"*Alimentary system.*—Tongue dry and coated, tip and edges clean. Bowels constipated. Appetite lost. Liver normal, no tenderness. Spleen is enlarged, no tenderness. Nausea and epigastric discomfort present.

"*Circulatory system.*—Heart sounds normal. Pulse slow and compressible, 98 per minute.

"*Respiratory system.*—Lungs normal, respirations hurried.

"*Urinary system.*—Patient passed six ounces of urine on admission. Examination: Acid reaction. Sp. gr. 1025. Albumen present.

"*Nervous system.*—Severe frontal headache. Aching pains in the loins and body. Reflexes normal.

"*Blood examination.*—No malaria parasites present. Leucopenia present. No pigmented leucocytes. Differential count: Polymorphonuclear, 76 per cent.; lymphocytes, 15·2 per cent.; mononuclear, 4·6 per cent.; eosinophil, 4·2 per cent.

"Temperature rose to 103·2° at 8 p.m., pulse rate 96.

"*16th May.*—Patient had a bad night, very restless and complained of severe headache and pains all over the body. No vomiting, but nausea present. Temperature at 8 a.m. was 102·4°, pulse rate 88. Urine passed, high in colour. Examination: Acid reaction. Sp. gr. 1020, albumen present.

"*17th May.*—Patient had a better night. Bowels opened. No vomiting. Headache and pains less. Urine passed, increased in quantity, albumen present, but lessened in amount. Temperature at 8 a.m. was 101·4°, pulse rate 78. Temperature rose towards evening and was 103·4° at 8 p.m., with a pulse rate of 84.

"*18th May.*—Patient had a quiet night, slept better. Headache and pains have gone. Bowels were opened freely. Urine passed in large quantity. Albumen still present, but lessened in amount. Conjunctivæ are now yellow. Appetite returning. Temperature still raised.

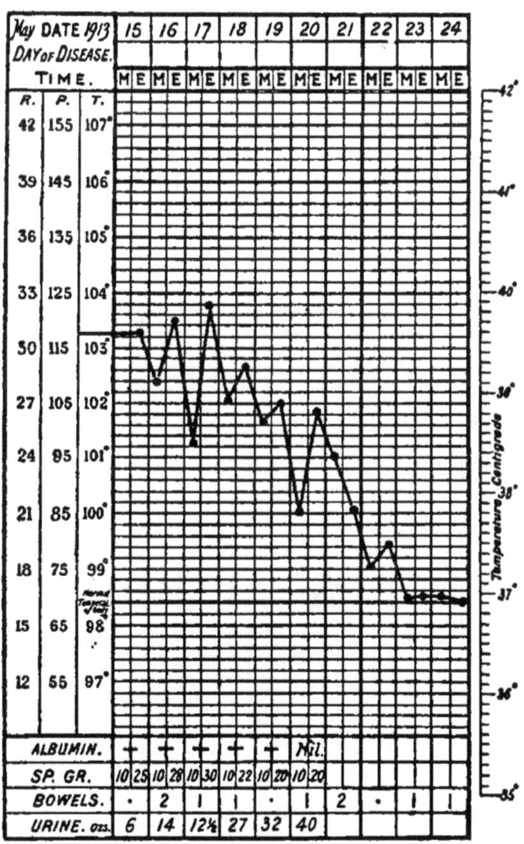

"Patient continued to improve daily, jaundice deepened Bowels became regular. Appetite increased. Urine increased in quantity and on the 20th May albumen disappeared from the urine and bile appeared.

"Patient made an uneventful recovery and was discharged cured on the 30th May."

The following case was classified as "Probable Yellow Fever":—

"Case No. 4. L. 24.

, Vol. I., 224-227.

"*Sex*: Male.
"*Age*: 22 years.
"*Nationality*: Negro, Yoruba tribe.
"*Occupation*: Sanitary inspector.
"*Date of admission*: 16th May, 1913.
"*Date of discharge*: 30th May, 1913.
"*Diagnosis*: Mild yellow fever.

"*History*.—Patient states that he began to feel ill about six days ago, the illness beginning with headache, rigors, and aching pains all over the body. He also had pyrexia. He continued at his work, but got worse, and reported sick and was sent to hospital.

"*On admission*.—Patient was admitted into hospital at 3.45 p.m. on the 16th May, complaining of fever, severe frontal headache and general aching pains. Bowels were also confined. He seemed very distressed. Conjunctivæ injected and red.

"*Alimentary system*.—Appetite lost. Bowels constipated. No vomiting. Nausea present. Tongue coated, with tip and edges clean. Liver normal. Spleen normal, no tenderness. No epigastralgia present, but this was present two days ago.

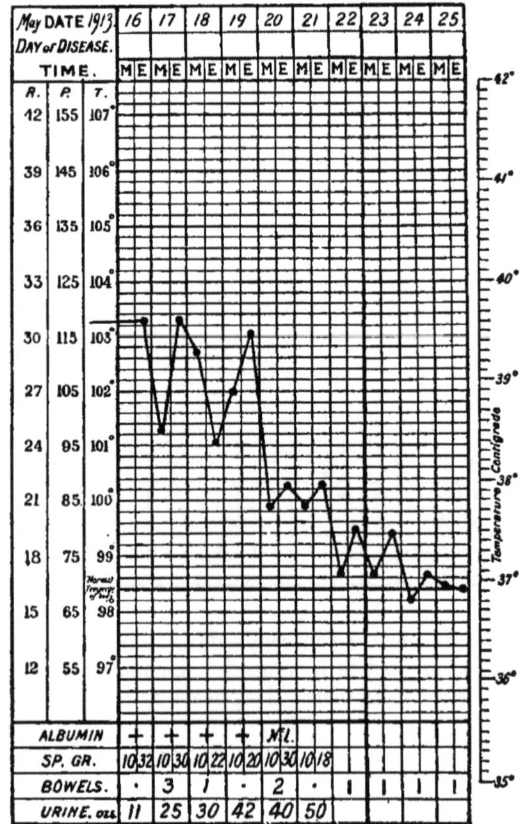

"*Circulatory system.*—Heart sounds normal. Pulse: low tension, 82 per minute.

"*Respiratory system.*—Lungs normal, respirations hurried.

"*Nervous system.*—Frontal headache and aching pains in the loins and extremities. Reflexes normal.

"*Urinary system.*—Patient had passed no urine since early morning and passed none after admission until 6 a.m. next day, the 17th. Examination: Reaction acid. Sp. gr. 1032. Albumen present.

"*Blood examination.*—No malaria parasites present. Leucopenia present. Differential count: Polymorphonuclear, 80 per cent.; mononuclear, 10 per cent.; lymphocytes, 10 per cent.

"Temperature on admission was 103·2°, pulse rate 82.

"*17th May.*—Patient had a very restless night, did not sleep. Temperature was raised, being 104° at 8 p.m., with a pulse of 82. Passed no urine during the night. Headache and pains were very severe. At 6 a.m. passed six ounces of very highly coloured urine which contained albumen. Temperature at 8 a.m. was 101·4°, pulse 84. Had an attack of vomiting, dark green fluid with brown debris. Temperature rose in the evening and at 8 p.m. was 103·4° with a pulse of 88. Bowels were opened twice.

"*18th May.*—Patient had a better night, is more comfortable and the headache and pains are lessened. Passed urine, but still diminished in quantity, high coloured and contains albumen. Temperature at 8 p.m. was 102·6°, pulse rate 88; at 8 p.m. temperature was 101°, pulse 84. Scleræ are now tinged with yellow.

"*19th May.*—Patient much better, had a better night. Bowels opened. No further vomiting. Urine increased in amount. Still contains albumen, but the percentage is lessened. Temperature at 8 a.m. was 102°, pulse rate 75. Temperature rose towards evening, and at 8 p.m. was 103·2°, pulse 88. Conjunctivæ are not so injected, scleræ are yellow.

"*20th May.*—Patient is very much better. Headache has quite gone. Bowels regular. Temperature falling. Urine has increased in amount and on examination is acid, sp. gr. 1020, no albumen present. Scleræ are very yellow. Appetite has improved.

"Patient continued to do well and slowly improved. Jaundice disappeared on the 26th May, and he was discharged from the hospital on the 30th May."

(*B*) SEVERE TYPE IN NATIVES.

Cases of the hæmorrhagic type in natives do not differ materially from those occurring in Europeans.

The following are examples of fatal cases in natives which were observed in the Freetown epidemic of 1910:—

5. ...eport. "A Negro, aged 23 years. By occupation a clerk on the railway.

"*Previous history*.—The patient had never been out of West Africa. His previous illnesses were not recorded. He had not been in the habit of taking quinine.

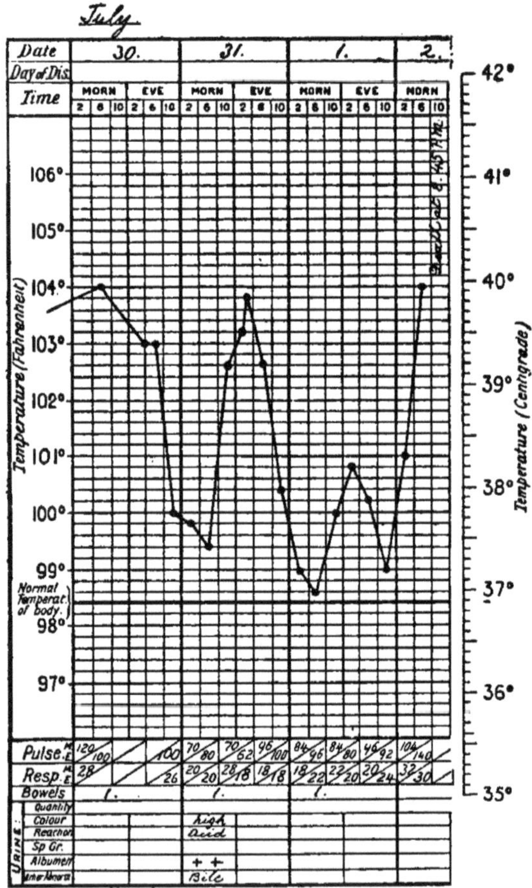

"*History of present illness*.—He stated that he had been ill since July 27th, suffering from fever and much pain in the back and chest; that he was treated as an out-patient and went home. On July 28th the previous symptoms were aggravated and he was unable to present

* The full reference is as follows:—"Report on Certain Outbreaks of Yellow Fever in 1910 and 1911." Waterlow & Sons Limited, London. (By A. E. Horn, M.D. and T. F. G. Mayer, M.R.C.S., L.R.C.P.) This Volume will be referred to thus: "Y.F. Report, p.—."

himself at the hospital for treatment as an out-patient. He was visited at home by his doctor. Throughout the day he vomited nearly all his food.

"On July 29th he was again visited by the doctor and admitted to hospital on July 30th when his temperature was 104°; he complained of pain in the abdomen, especially in the hepatic area. His general condition was weak. He stated that vomiting was troublesome, and that the vomited matter was of a yellowish green colour and liquid. The bowels were freely opened. The pulse rate was 120; the respirations 28; the tongue was coated; the eyes were jaundiced. At 10 p.m. the temperature was 103°.

"On July 31st at 6 a.m. the patient felt a great deal better. He had slept fairly well and the temperature was 99·4°. The pain in the chest and abdomen was a little better than on the previous day. The urine was highly coloured, there was much deposit in it. Its specific gravity was 1025, it was acid in reaction, highly albuminous, and bile was present in it.

"The patient was delirious and somewhat restless during the night.

"On August 1st at 6 a.m. the temperature was normal. The patient was very weak. The eyes were very much jaundiced. The urine was highly coloured and contained much deposit. He vomited the medicine given him once during the day, and passed one motion of a yellow colour.

"He was somewhat delirious during the night and passed his urine into his bed.

"He looked very weak and restless on the morning of August 2nd. At 6 a.m. the temperature was 104°, the pulse 140 and the respiration 30. A hypodermic injection of digitalin and strychnine was given; at 8.45 a.m. the patient died in convulsion, the temperature being 104°.

"No microscopical blood examination was made during the patient's illness.

"*Post-mortem examination.*—A limited examination only was allowed.

"The stomach contained 'coffee-grounds.' A portion near the cardiac end was marked with arborescent and congested capillaries.

"The liver was of a typical boxwood colour."

"A Negro Labourer of the Mendi tribe, aged about 26 years, living in Freetown (Kru-bay). Case 20. Y.F Report, p. 42.

"*Previous history.*—He was a native of Sierra Leone. His previous illnesses had not been recorded. He had not been in the habit of taking quinine. He had not been out of Freetown for some time before the present illness.

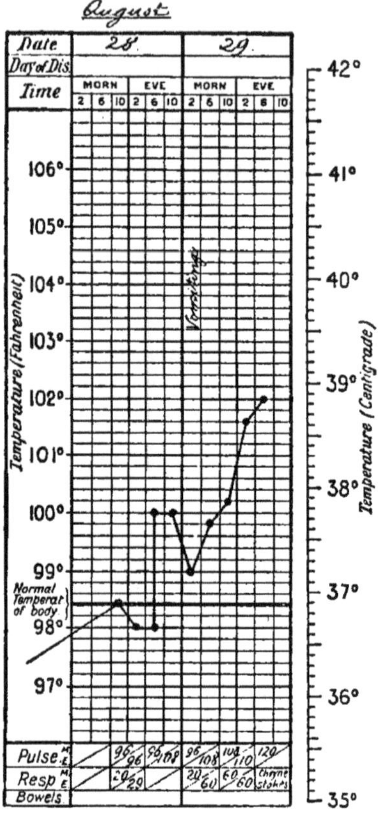

"*History of present illness.*—On August 28th, at 6.30 p.m., the patient was admitted to hospital. He was said to have been taken ill three days before with fever, headache and pains all over his body. His skin was cold and his pulse weak. He was restless, tossing about so much that his temperature could not be taken; the pupils were dilated and did not react to light. He appeared stupefied, but could be roused. There was retention of urine and the bladder was distended. A soft catheter was passed and drew off ten ounces of urine.

"On August 29th he had black vomit in the morning. His condition resembled that of the day before. He was very weak. The temperature was 97·8°, the pulse 96, respirations 20 to the minute. In the afternoon he again vomited. His skin was cold and clammy, that of the face was perspiring freely. His condition did not improve, his temperature rising to 101·8°. At 6.45 p.m. the patient died.

"*Post-mortem examination.*—The lungs: There was considerable œdema of the left lung.

"The stomach contained a large quantity of black fluid like that which was vomited, and there were punctate hæmorrhages in the mucous membrane of the stomach wall.

"The small intestines also contained much black fluid like that in the stomach.

"The liver was mottled.

"The kidneys were congested, there were hæmorrhages under the capsule.

"The brain was congested, but there were no hæmorrhages into it."

(*c*) MILD TYPE IN EUROPEANS.

The following is an example of a case of the mild type in a European. It was classified by the Commission as "Probable Yellow Fever."

"Case No. 2.—Lagos. L. 122.

"*Sex*: Male.

"*Age*: 27 years.

"*Nationality*: European, German.

"*Occupation*: Trader.

"*Date of admission*: 14th February, 1914.

"*Date of discharge*: 27th February, 1914.

"*Diagnosis*: Yellow fever.

"*History.*—Patient states that he felt ill yesterday, the 13th, in the morning, with chills and frontal headache. Became gradually worse during the day, and at night his temperature was 104°, with very severe headache and pains in the extremities. He was seen by his medical attendant, Dr. Maples, who gave him an intramuscular injection of quinine. He had a bad night, but felt better early next morning. During the day the temperature again rose, headache became severe, nausea and epigastric discomfort was present. No vomiting until he made himself vomit to relieve the nausea. In the evening his temperature was 104°, conjunctivæ were injected and red, headache very severe, and his urine on examination was albuminous. So he was sent to the hospital at 7 p.m.

"*On admission.*—Temperature was 101·8°, pulse rate 98. Conjunctivæ very injected. Complained of severe frontal headache and aching pains in the loins. Patient has only been out eight months of this, his first, tour. Has taken quinine regularly.

"*Alimentary system.*—Gums red and swollen. Tongue, white dorsum, with red tip and edges. Bowels constipated. Liver and spleen both normal, no tenderness. Nausea and epigastric discomfort present. Great thirst present.

"*Circulatory system.*—Heart sounds normal. Pulse slow, 90 at 8 p.m.

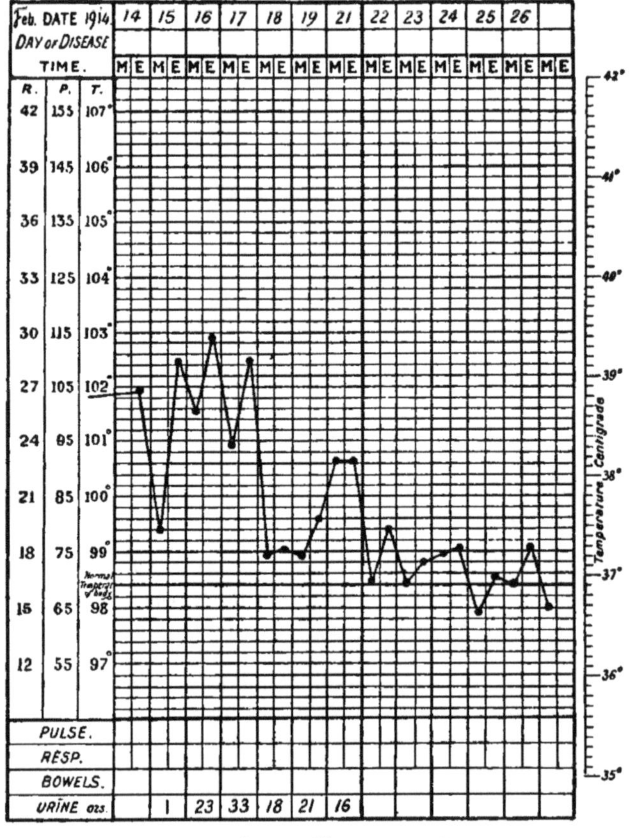

"*Respiratory system.*— Lungs normal. Respirations hurried.

"*Nervous system.*—Severe frontal headache present. Aching pains in the loins. Reflexes normal.

"*Urinary system.*—Urine passed on admission. Very high coloured. Acid reaction. Sp. gr. 1030. Albumen present, high percentage. Quantity has been diminished.

"*Other systems.*—Skin, sweating. Face very flushed. Conjunctivæ injected. Eyes shining. Photophobia present.

"*Blood examination.*—No malaria parasites present. *Paraplasma flavigenum* present. Differential count: Polymorphonuclears, 61 per cent.; lymphocytes, 27·4 per cent.; mononuclear, 8·4 per cent.; transitionals, 2·8 per cent.; mast cells, 0·4 per cent.

"*15th February.*—Patient had a fair night, but was restless in the early part. Bowels moved after calomel. Urine passed, but diminished in quantity, only 7 ozs. passed in the previous twenty-four hours. Highly albuminous. Temperature at 8 a.m. was 99·4°, pulse rate 88. Tube casts present in the urine. During the day the temperature rose, and at 4 p.m. was 103·6°, pulse 100. Patient very excitable, complained of great thirst. Face very flushed and conjunctivæ were very injected. At 8 p.m. temperature was 102·4°, pulse 96.

"*16th February.*—Patient was very restless last night and only slept after a draught. Conjunctivæ very injected. Nausea troublesome. Urine still diminished and contains albumen. Patient is very nervous and complains of great thirst. Temperature at 8 a.m. was 101·6°, pulse rate 88. At 8 p.m. temperature rose to 102·8°, pulse rate 90.

"*17th February.*—Patient had a better night and slept. Is feeling much improved this morning. Temperature at 8 a.m. 100·6°, pulse 100. Headache still present, also loin pains. Urine is still diminished and contains albumen, sp. gr. 1030, acid reaction. At 8 p.m. temperature rose to 102·4°, with pulse of 90. Thirst is lessened. Conjunctivæ still injected.

"*18th February.*—Patient had a good night and is feeling very much better. Bowels opened. Urine passed in increased quantity, and on examination still contains albumen. Conjunctival injection passing off. Scleræ are now tinged with yellow. Temperature is 99°, with pulse rate of 100.

"*19th February.*—Patient is much improved and had a good night. Temperature still 99°. Bowels opened. Urine examined and found to contain bile, but no albumen. Scleræ are decidedly yellow. Nausea and epigastric discomfort have passed off. Appetite is returning. Urine has not yet reached the normal. Headache quite gone.

"Patient continued to improve gradually, jaundice slowly disappeared on the 24th, and patient was discharged cured on the 27th February.

"NOTE BY COMMISSION.

"Some blood films from this case were examined by Dr. Wenyon, who found red cells with patches of basophilic change. In one film curious star-like artefacts occurred which he thought might be mistaken for parasites."

(*d*) SEVERE TYPE IN EUROPEANS.

The following case occurred in the Lagos epidemic of 1913:—

"CASE NO. 7. L. 37.

"*Sex*: Male.

"*Age*: 34.

"*Nationality*: European, British.

"*Occupation*: Bank accountant.

"*Date of admission*: 17th July, 1913.

"*Date of death*: 20th July, 1913.

"*Diagnosis*: Yellow fever.

"*History*.—Patient states that on the 16th he began to feel ill about mid-day with chilly sensations, followed by frontal headache. He finished his work and in the evening had to go to bed as he was feeling worse. The headache had increased in severity and he had racking pains in the loins and limbs. He was seen by a doctor that night, and also next morning, and as his condition seemed serious he was sent into hospital.

"Patient has had several attacks of malarial fever. Present tour in Lagos 7½ months' duration. Has kept good health up to the present.

"*On admission*.—Patient complains of great and severe frontal and ocular headache with racking pains in the loins and extremities. Face is flushed, conjunctivæ injected and the eyes shining and watery. Bowels have been confined, nausea is present, and he has pain and discomfort in the epigastrium, increasing on pressure.

"*Alimentary system*.—Bowels are constipated, appetite lost. Tongue is pointed, with red tip and edges and furred dorsum. Liver is normal, no tenderness. Spleen is also normal. Epigastrium is tender and painful on pressure.

"*Circulatory system*.—Heart sounds are normal. Pulse is slow, low tension, 96 per minute.

"*Respiratory system*.—Lungs normal. Respirations hurried.

"*Nervous system*.—Severe frontal headache and pains in the eyes. Racking pains in the loins and extremities. Reflexes normal.

"*Urinary system*.—Urine is very cloudy and diminished. Examination: Acid. Sp. gr. 1022. Albumen present.

"*Blood examination*.—No malaria parasites present. Pigmented leucocytes present. *Paraplasma flavigenum* present. Differential count: Polymorphonuclear, 78 per cent.; mononuclear, 7 per cent.; lymphocytes, 13 per cent.; eosinophil, 2 per cent. Leucopenia present.

"Temperature on admission at 10 p.m. was 103·8°, pulse rate 96.

"*18th July*.—Patient had a quiet night, headache not so severe this morning. Eyes injected and shining. At 8 a.m. temperature was 104°, with a pulse rate of 80. About 10 a.m. patient felt uncomfortable in the stomach and caused himself to vomit. Vomited matter consisted of a dark brown fluid with chocolate-coloured debris. Bowels moved at 10.30 a.m., motion being a greenish fluid with chocolate-coloured debris. Vomiting stopped after the application of a sinapism, but nausea and gastric discomfort were present. Temperature at 104° all the evening and at 8 p.m. was 104·4°, pulse rate 70. Bowels were again moved at 8 p.m. and the motions contained dark chocolate-coloured debris. Passed eight ounces of very muddy urine, which contained a large amount of albumen.

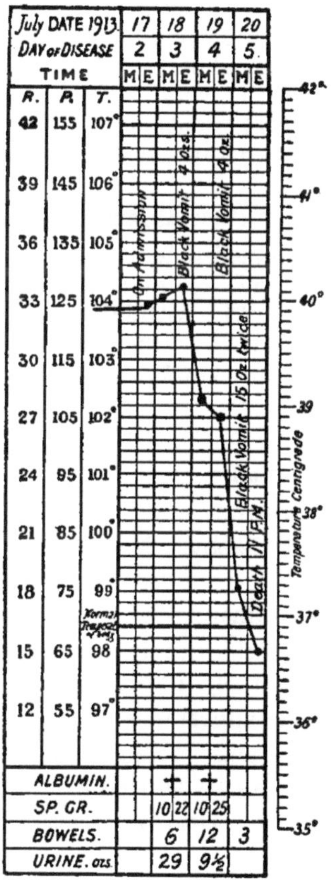

July DATE 1913.	17		18		19		20	
DAY OF DISEASE	2		3		4		5	
TIME	M	E	M	E	M	E	M	E
ALBUMIN.			+		+			
SP. GR.			10	22	10	25		
BOWELS.			6		12		3	
URINE. ozs.			29		9½			

R.	P.	T.
42	155	107°
39	145	106°
36	135	105°
33	125	104°
30	115	103°
27	105	102°
24	95	101°
21	85	100°
18	75	99°
15	65	98°
12	55	97°

On Admission
Black Vomit 4 Ozs.
Black Vomit 4 Oz.
Black Vomit 15 Oz. twice
Death 11 P.M.
Normal Temperature
Temperature Centigrade: 42°, 41°, 40°, 39, 38°, 37°, 36°, 35°

"*19th July.*—Patient had a restless night and did not get much sleep. During the early hours of the morning patient had several motions and the stools were dark and chocolate-coloured. Eyes were still injected. Epigastric pain and discomfort with nausea present. An erythematous rash appeared on the skin of neck and chest. Urine was diminished and contained a large percentage of albumen. Temperature at 8 a.m. was 102·4°, pulse rate 64. In the afternoon, at 5.20 p.m., patient had an attack of vomiting, four ounces of black vomit. Bowels moved again and the stools were black and tarry. No urine passed except the one ounce at 1 p.m. Black vomit again occurred at 7.15 p.m. and petechial hæmorrhages appeared in the skin of neck, chest and back. The temperature at 8 p.m. was 101·8°, pulse rate 68. Only 1½ ounces of urine passed in the twelve hours.

"*20th July.*—Patient had a fair night and was quieter. Bowels moved several times towards morning; the stools were black and tarry. No more vomiting during the night, but at 8.40 a.m. he had a severe attack and vomited 12 ounces of black vomit. No urine was passed through the night. Skin was jaundiced. Temperature 101·4°, pulse rate 68. Conjunctivæ showed small hæmorrhages and the scleræ was deeply jaundiced. Patient became much worse towards the evening. Very restless, with subsultus tendinum very marked. Ecchymoses of the genital organs very pronounced. Urine suppressed. Delirium present. Vomiting became almost continuous, typical black vomit. Patient's condition became very serious, skin deeply jaundiced, petechial hæmorrhages more pronounced. Very restless and delirious. At 10 p.m. convulsions set in and lasted for about an hour, and death occurred at 11 p.m.

"POST-MORTEM NOTES.

"Autopsy was performed nine hours after death.

"Rigor mortis present. Skin deeply jaundiced. Post-mortem staining of dependent parts. Genital organs cyanosed. Palms of hands and soles of feet stained a deep yellow. Petechial hæmorrhages in skin of neck, back and chest. Subconjunctival hæmorrhages in both eyes.

"*Brain.*—Normal. No congestion.

"*Spinal cord.*—Normal.

"*Membranes.*—Normal.

"*Heart.*—Pale and flabby. Valves normal. No hæmorrhages. Weight, 8½ ounces.

"*Large vessels.*—Normal.

"*Lung, right.*—Bronchi deeply congested. Base of lung congested and areas of hæmorrhage present.

"*Lung, left.*—Same appearance as right.

"*Pleuræ.*—No adhesions present. Each cavity contained four ounces of yellow fluid. No hæmorrhages.

"*Larynx and trachea.*—Deeply congested.

"*Peritoneum.*—Normal.

"*Oesophagus.*—Intensely congested.

"*Stomach.*—Contained ten ounces of black fluid. Mucous membrane congested. Rugæ swollen and thrown into corrugations. Patches of hæmorrhage in mucous membrane, most marked at the cardiac end and along the lesser curvature. Large hæmorrhage in posterior wall.

"*Small intestine.*—Duodenum intensely congested. Submucous hæmorrhages along its entire length. Jejunum also congested and hæmorrhages present. Ileum congested for about half its length. The intestinal canal contained a dark, tarry fluid.

"*Large intestine.*—Mucous membrane congested and gelatinous in appearance near the ileo-cæcal valve. Empty.

"*Helminths.*—None present.

"*Liver.*—Pale, boxwood colour. No hæmorrhages in capsule. On section, greasy. Very friable. Weight, 58½ ounces.

"*Gall bladder.*—Empty. Mucous membrane congested.

"*Pancreas.*—Normal. Weight, 5 ounces.

"*Spleen.*—Slightly enlarged and congested. Weight, 7½ ounces.

"*Kidney, right.*—Enlarged. Capsule strips easily. Dilated stellate veins under capsule. Weight, 8½ ounces.

"*Kidney, left.*—Enlarged. Capsule strips easily. Weight, 8 ounces.

"*Suprarenal capsules.*—Normal.

"*Lymphatic system.*—Normal.

"*Bladder.*—Contracted and contained ¼ ounce of very dark brown urine. Highly albuminous on examination. Mucous membrane normal.

"LABORATORY REPORT.

"*Microscopic examination:*

"Blood smears showed no malaria parasites.

"*Histological examination:*

"*Liver.*—Advanced fatty degeneration. Cells vacuolated and protoplasm granular. Distorted arrangement of lobules.

"*Kidney.*—Cells swollen and granular. Tubules denuded of epithelium in places and filled with granular and hyaline debris. Droplets of fat in cells of convoluted tubules. Several small hæmorrhages.

"*Stomach.*—Mucous membrane swollen and vessels congested. Punctiform hæmorrhages present.

"*Spleen.*—Congested. Capsule thickened."

The following is an example of a fatal case in a Syrian:—

"CASE NO. 11. L. 41.

"*Sex*: Male.

"*Age*: 35 years.

"*Nationality*: Syrian.

"*Occupation*: Trader.

"*Date of admission*: 25th July, 1913.

"*Date of death*: 28th July, 1913.

"*Diagnosis*: Yellow Fever.

"*History.*—Patient was admitted into hospital at 9 p.m. on the 25th July from the Isolation Hospital, where he had been under observation from the 20th. He was one of the occupants of the house in which Case No. 8 had occurred, and had been removed with the other contacts on the 20th. On the morning of the 24th he complained of not feeling well, and that he had a severe headache and aching pains in the back and limbs. In the evening his temperature rose and he had vomiting, bilious in character. He had a restless night and was much worse next day, and was sent to the Lagos Hospital.

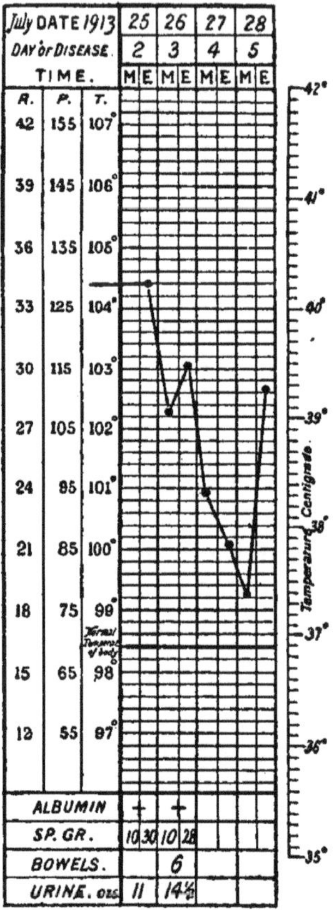

"*On admission.*—Patient was very distressed, respirations were hurried. Face was flushed, eyes shining and bright. Conjunctivæ were very injected and red. Temperature 104·6°, pulse rate 120 per minute.

"*Alimentary system.*—Appetite lost. Bowels constipated. Tongue dry and pointed, with white dorsum and red tip and edges. Liver was normal, no tenderness. Spleen was enlarged and palpable, no tenderness. Nausea was present, with epigastric pain and discomfort, which increased on pressure.

"*Circulatory system.*—Heart sounds normal. Pulse 120 per minute.

"*Respiratory system.*—Lungs normal. Respirations hurried.

"*Urinary system.*—Patient passed 2 ozs. of urine after admission. Examination: Acid reaction. Sp. gr. 1030. Albumen present, high percentage.

"*Blood examination.*—No malaria parasites present. *Paraplasma flavigenum* present. Pigmented leucocytes present. Differential count: Polymorphonuclear, 76 per cent.; mononuclear, 7 per cent.; lymphocytes, 13 per cent.; eosinophil, 4 per cent.

"Temperature rose at 10 p.m. to 104·4°, pulse rate 112.

"*26th July.*—Patient had a bad night, very restless. Complained of severe frontal headache and pains in the loins. At 8 a.m. temperature was 102·4°, with a pulse rate of 90. Had an attack of vomiting, bilious in character. Passed 14 ozs. of urine, which on examination was found to be highly albuminous. Temperature rose in the afternoon and at 8 p.m. it was 103·2°, with a pulse of 84. Patient is looking very ill. Conjunctivæ very injected and red. Epigastric pain and discomfort, with nausea present. Vomited several times during the afternoon.

"*27th July.*—Patient had a bad night, very restless. No urine passed at all. Temperature at 8 a.m. was 100·8°, pulse rate 72. Vomited at 8.30 a.m. a clear fluid with chocolate-coloured debris. Scleræ are yellow. Nausea still present with epigastric discomfort.

"*28th July.*—Patient passed a quiet night. No urine passed for the past twenty-four hours. Temperature at 8 a.m. was 99·4°, pulse rate 72. Temperature began to rise in the afternoon and at 8 p.m. was 102·6°. Patient began to get comatose, and death occurred quietly at 8.15 p.m. Skin deeply jaundiced.

"POST-MORTEM NOTES.

"Autopsy was performed twelve hours after death.

"Rigor mortis present.

"Skin and scleræ stained an intense yellow. Genital organs cyanosed.

"*Brain.*—Appeared normal.

"*Spinal cord.*—Normal.

"*Membranes.*—Congested.

"*Pericardium.*—Showed old adhesions. Contained 1 oz. of fluid.

"*Heart.*—Pale and flabby. Minute hæmorrhages seen on the surface of the ventricles. Valves normal. Sub-endocardial hæmorrhages well marked in the left ventricle. Weight, 8½ ozs.

"*Large vessels.*—Normal.

"*Lung, right.*—Very congested, particularly at base.

"*Lung, left.*—Same as right.

"*Pleuræ.*—Adhesions present in right side, left side normal. Some effusion present.

"*Larynx and trachea.*—Normal.

"*Peritoneum.*—Normal.

"*Stomach.*—Contents 10 ozs. of black fluid. Mucous membrane very congested. Rugæ swollen and prominent. Submucous hæmorrhages well marked at the cardiac and pyloric ends. Large extensive hæmorrhage along the greater curvature.

"*Small intestine.*—Duodenum intensely congested. Numerous submucous hæmorrhages present. Contained black fluid similar to that in the stomach. Jejunum also intensely congested and minute submucous hæmorrhages present. Ileum very congested along its entire length to within two feet of the ileo-cæcal valve.

"*Large intestine.*—Mucous membrane congested and thickened. Contents a brown fluid.

"*Helminths.*—Numerous ascarides Two tape worms (*T. saginata*) also found.

"*Liver.*—Pale yellow in appearance with patches of hyperæmia. Well marked subcapsular hæmorrhages. On section, greasy and very friable. Weight, 46 ozs.

"*Gall bladder.*—Normal.

"*Pancreas.*—Normal. Weight, 5 ozs.

"*Spleen.*—Enlarged and tough. Congested. Weight, 14½ ozs.

"*Kidney, right.*—Very congested. Enlarged. Capsule strips easily. On section, cortex congested, medullary portion showing hæmorrhages. Weight, 6½ ozs.

"*Kidney, left.*—Same as the right. Weight, 7 ozs.

"*Suprarenal capsules.*—Normal appearance.

"*Lymphatic system.*—Normal.

"*Bladder.*—Contracted. Contained 1 oz. of dark, turbid urine. Acid reaction and highly albuminous.

"LABORATORY REPORT.

"*Histological.*

"*Liver.*—Profound fatty degeneration present. Great increase of fibrous tissue. Normal structure of organ practically obliterated. The few cells clearly visible contained fatty globules and vacuoles.

"*Kidney.*—Hyperæmia and a number of hæmorrhages present. Cells of the convoluted tubules were swollen and granular. Tubules denuded in places, and filled with granular and hyaline debris.

"*Spleen.*—Engorged.

"*Stomach and intestines.*—Ecchymoses present. Vessels engorged. Epithelium swollen and granular."

The consideration of the clinical features of the various types is reserved for the section on "Diagnosis" (*vide* pp. 153-159).

SECTION IX.

SYMPTOMATOLOGY.

To discuss in detail the symptomatology of such a disease as Yellow Fever would result in the production of a bulky text book, and is obviously beyond the scope of this report and of the reference to the Commission.

Moreover, the cases constituting the epidemics of 1910 and 1911 at Freetown, Seccondee, Saw Mills, Axim, Lagos, Accra and Bathurst have already been analysed very fully by Drs. Horn and Mayer, who were in succession attached to the Colonial Office, about that period, and the results are contained in the "Report on Certain Outbreaks of Yellow Fever in 1910 and 1911," issued by the Colonial Office in 1913 (*vide* pp. 88-91).

Dr. E. J. Wyler has analysed, under similar headings, the cases occurring at Lagos in 1913 and 1914 (*vide* I.R., Vol. I., pp. 142-144), and Dr. Leonard has also submitted those cases to a very careful analysis, which will be found in the same volume of the Reports by Investigators (*vide* pp. 291-294).

The synopsis of those cases emphasises the statements in the Second Report as to the infinite variety in which Yellow Fever may present itself even in a single epidemic, a lesson learned from a careful reading of the "Report on the Pathology, Therapeutics, and general Aitology of the epidemic of Yellow Fever which prevailed at Lisbon during the latter half of the year 1857, by Dr. Robert D. Lyons, late Pathologist in the Crimea." That report, as already stated, probably contains the most masterly description of the disease to be found in all the mass of literature on the subject of Yellow Fever. If the complex of symptoms which constitutes the disease is subject to this degree of variation in a single epidemic, it is seen to be infinitely more varied when successive outbreaks are considered, and an attempt is made to construct from the records of the cases a clinical picture of the disease.

We must be content to refer the reader to those analyses and clinical reports, in which he will see that certain symptoms which are emphasized in the Section on Diagnosis (*vide* p. 152) stand out as landmarks, and that on these attention must be concentrated when a doubtful case is under consideration.

(*A*) PYREXIA.

The remission of the fever which often occurs on the third day or later, gives to the temperature chart the typical "saddle-back" character, but this feature is by no means constant, and it may be of service to illustrate, by charts of cases which have been observed, the types of pyrexia most often met with.

(I) REMITTENT TYPE (RECOVERY).

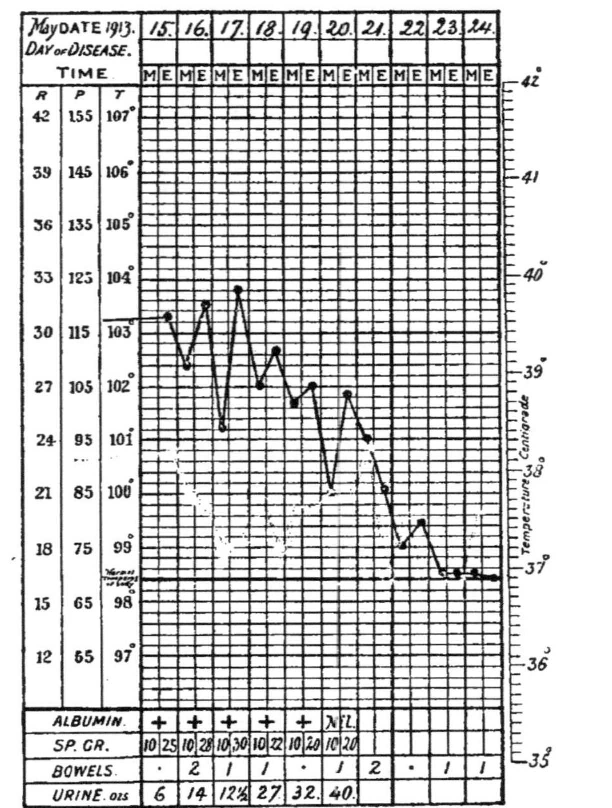

Case No. 3, L. 25. p. 225. I.R., Vol. I.

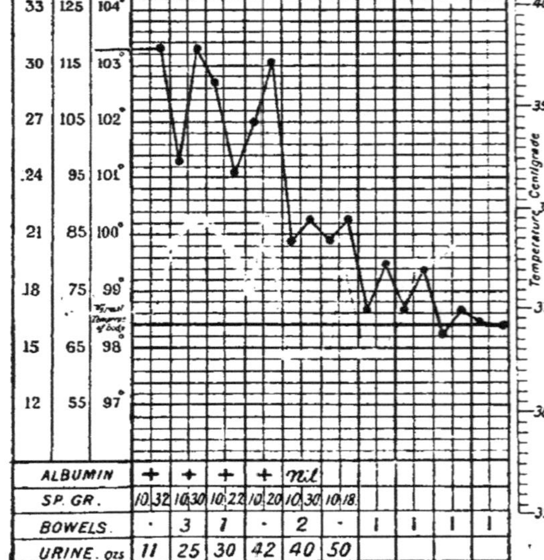

Case No. 4, I., 24. p. 226. I.R., Vol. I.

(II) REMITTENT OR SADDLE-BACK TYPE (FATAL).

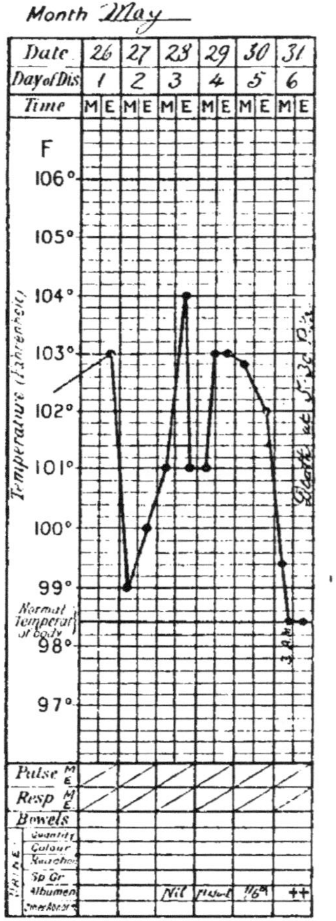

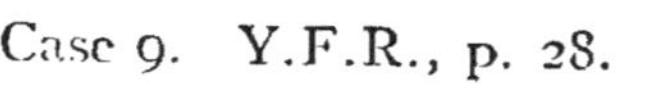

Case 9. Y.F.R., p. 28.

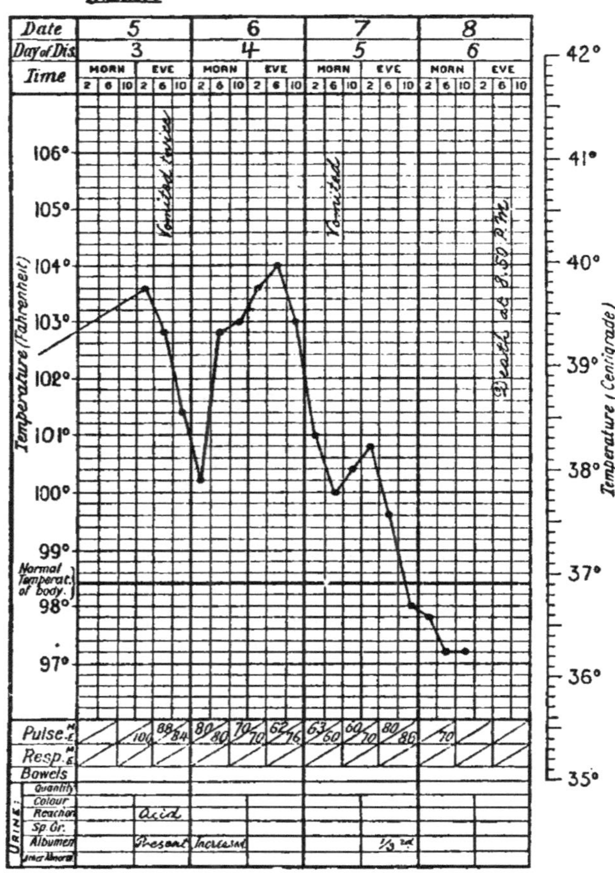

Case 10. Y.F.R., p. 29.

(II) REMITTENT OR SADDLE-BACK TYPE (FATAL)—
continued.

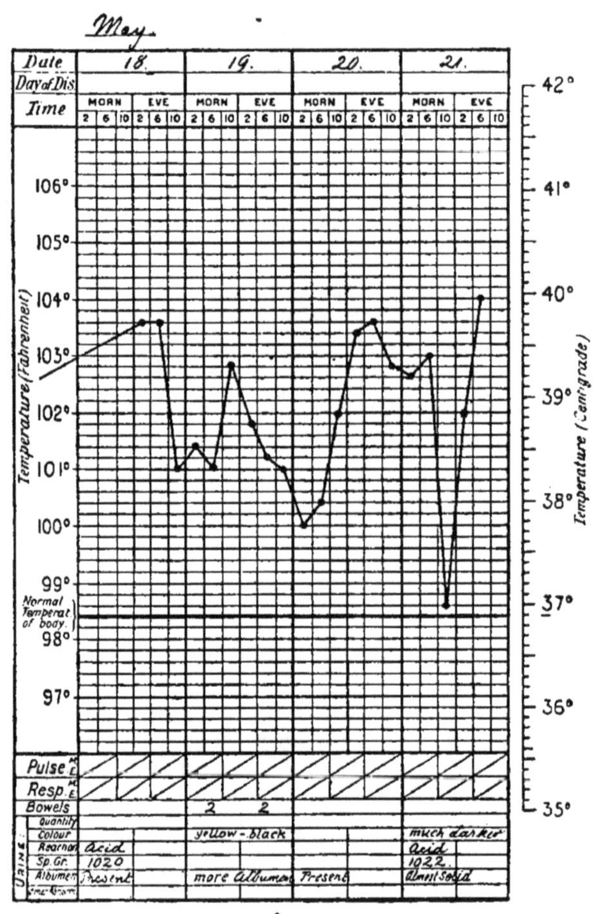

Case 30. Y.F.R., p. 52.

(III) DESCENDING TYPE.

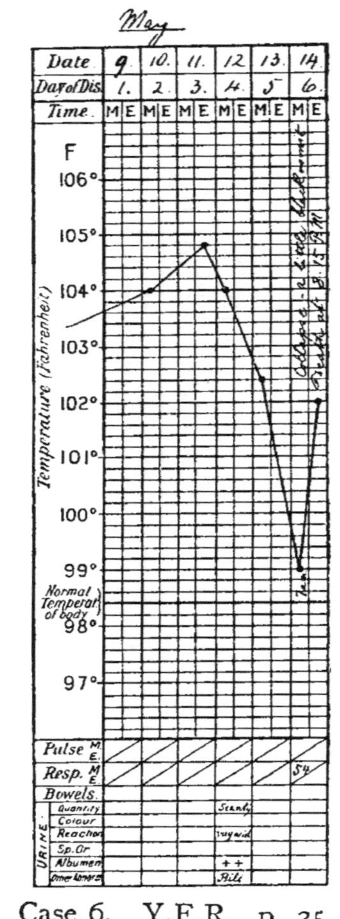

Case 6. Y.F.R., p. 25.

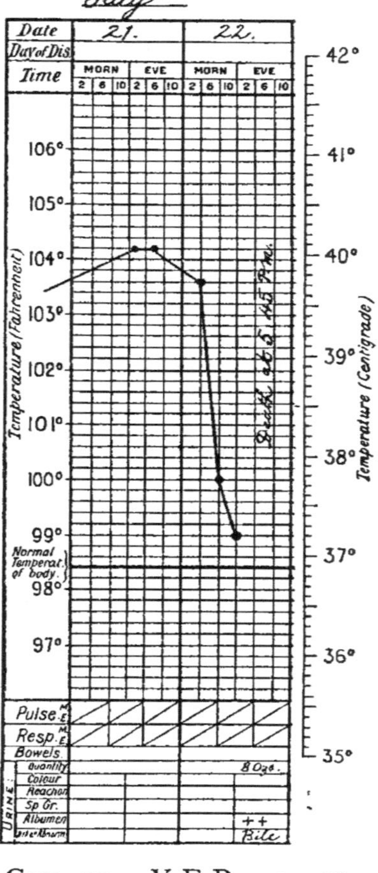

Case 13. Y.F.R., p. 35.

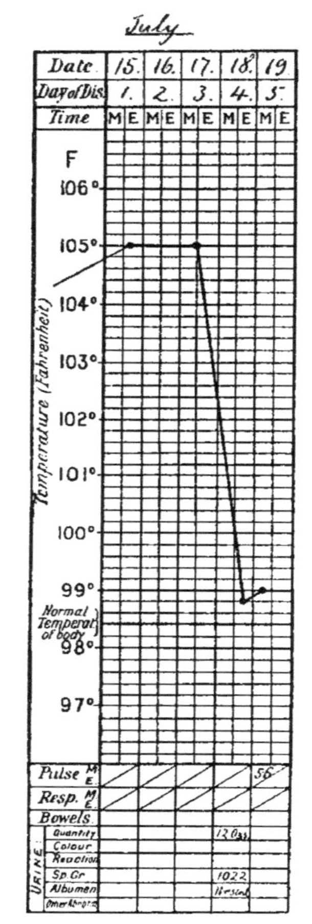

Case 35. Y.F.R., p. 57.

(IV) CONTINUED TYPE (WITH SLIGHT REMISSIONS).

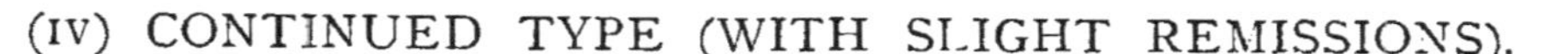

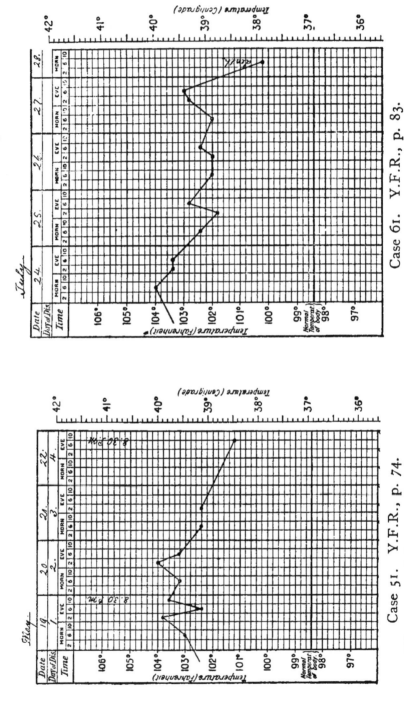

Case 51. Y.F.R., p. 74.

Case 61. Y.F.R., p. 83.

The nature of the cases attended with hyperpyrexia is separately considered (*vide* p. 188).

(*B*) THE CHARACTER AND COURSE OF THE JAUNDICE.

The jaundice of Yellow Fever is probably of hæmatogenous origin and not due to biliary obstruction, otherwise the fæces should be clay coloured, a condition which is rarely observed. The skin is at first of a pale yellow tinge, later of a deep orange colour, and this may deepen into a dark mahogany brown. The time of its appearance is dealt with in the section on Diagnosis (*vide* p. 152). After the scleræ it is seen in the skin of the face, neck and upper part of the trunk, and if absent during life, as it may be, it is almost invariably developed after death. During convalescence it gradually disappears.

The association of jaundice with malaria of the bilious remittent type is considered on page 161.

(*C*) THE CHARACTER OF THE VOMITED MATTERS.

It may be of interest to record the successive changes observed in the character of the vomited matters in some fatal cases.

Case 1.—A European:—

(*a*) Pale, greenish fluid with dark chocolate-coloured debris.
(*b*) Greenish fluid with chocolate-coloured debris.
(*c*) Thick dark brown fluid.
(*d*) Black vomit.

Case 2.—A European:—

(*a*) Dark brown fluid with chocolate-coloured debris.
(*b*) Black vomit.

Case 3.—A Syrian —:

(*a*) Colourless fluid with chocolate-coloured debris.
(*b*) Black vomit.

Case 4:—

(*a*) Bilious.
(*b*) A clear fluid with chocolate-coloured debris.
(*c*) Black fluid.

Case 5.—A Syrian:—

(*a*) Dark green fluid.
(*b*) Almost black fluid.

Case 6.—A European:—

(*a*) Bile.
(*b*) Dark green fluid.
(*c*) Black fluid.
(*d*) "Black vomit," followed by
(*e*) Dark blood.

Case 7.—A European:—

(*a*) Dark "coffee ground" material.
(*b*) A very dark stringy black coffee ground material.

Case 8.—A native:—

(*a*) All food taken.
(*b*) Yellowish green liquid.
(*c*) Coffee grounds.

The occurrence of the appearance usually described as "fly specks" in the vomit, which may precede the onset of true black vomit, is recorded in the following case:—

Case 9.—A European:—

(*a*) The vomit contained black specks.
(*b*) "Vomited a large quantity of black matter and died."

It is to be noted that all these cases were fatal, but that in the earlier stages the vomited matter did not present the appearance which some are disposed to regard as alone typical of Yellow Fever, *i.e.*, "black vomit."

We may recall what is stated in the Second Report (p. 66) to have occurred in the French Soudan in the years 1887 and 1888:—

"'Typho-malarial Fever' continued, but was of a less severe type. In discussing the nature of these epidemics it is mentioned that 'the errors in diagnosis' were due to the absence of 'black vomit' in more than half the cases, owing to the fact that the patients died before there had been time for the appearance of this symptom. Epistaxis and tarry stools were, however, noted in some of these cases. The conclusion is arrived at that, under various names, the disease throughout was Yellow Fever, and that there had been an annual epidemic from 1878 to 1888."

SECTION X.

DIAGNOSIS.

The diagnosis of Yellow Fever is a problem for the clinician and often a very difficult one. When he is in doubt the laboratory does not come to his aid, and, perhaps for his own good, he has to depend upon his powers of observation. For his comfort we may recall (*vide* Second Report, p. 110) Dr. Kohnke's observation that "Diagnosticians who can at all times differentiate between the very mild cases of Yellow Fever and diseases resembling it, exist mainly in the imagination of the laity."

Whatever difficulties may arise when we attempt to determine the nature of a suspected case of this disease from the perusal of a written record, we doubt whether at the bed-side they are sensibly greater than those which attended the diagnosis of, say, Enteric Fever before the introduction of the Widal test, or of certain other diseases in the pre-laboratory period. The physician who does not commence his examination of any and every patient by a prolonged look at his face is apt to miss much that the eye trained by many years of clinical experience can see at a glance, and is likely to be numbered with those who are paralysed when the resources of a clinical laboratory are not available.

The Commission has fortunately had the advantage of seeing physicians from abroad whose views on this and other problems of the enquiry have been formed as the result of such an experience, and at these interviews the important question of the diagnosis of the disease has not been overlooked.

The recognition of this, as of many other diseases, depends upon the capacity to observe and to attach the true value to the presence or absence of each one of a number of separate features, and not upon the presence or absence of some one of their number. In other words, no single sign or symptom is characteristic, or pathognomonic of Yellow Fever, each may in turn be absent; the disease is to be recognised from the clinical picture viewed as a whole.

(*A*) DIAGNOSIS OF CASES OF THE MILD TYPE.

The most important signs and symptoms are as follows:—

1. *The Aspect of the Patient.*—There is a degree of distress out of proportion to the temperature and to the urgency of the other symptoms. Insomnia, troubled sleep and *restlessness* are very often observed.

In the recorded cases, the following statements constantly recur.

"The patient was in great distress."

"The patient had a very anxious and distressed appearance."

"Patient was very distressed and looked ill."

"He felt very ill and had to go to bed."

2. *Flushing of the Face and Injection of the Conjunctivæ.*—There is an intense active capillary congestion of the skin and mucous membranes. The eyes are bloodshot and watery; the face is red and swollen; the upper lip is often puffy.

3. *Severe Frontal Headache.*—This symptom is rarely absent and usually attends the onset. The headache of Yellow Fever is almost invariably frontal, and it is very probable that the great distress and restlessness just described are in great part due to the intensely severe headache.

4. *Aching pains* in the loins and limbs and elsewhere.

Pains of this nature are, of course, common at the onset in many febrile diseases, particularly Influenza, but in Yellow Fever they are specially severe, and out of proportion to the pyrexia.

The following descriptions are typical:—

"Aches and pains all over the body."

"Aching pains in the loins and all over the body."

"Pains and aches all over the body, especially in the loins."

"Racking pains in the loins and extremities."

"Aching pains in the back and extremities."

5. *Epigastric Tenderness.*—This is generally recognised as a very common and an important symptom; it was noted as present in 22 out of 38 cases in the Lagos epidemic.

Dr. Paez (*vide* p. 162) lays special stress upon *Epigastric pulsation* as of great importance in diagnosis.

6. On or about the third day in cases of this type the aspect of the patient changes, the stage of *restlessness* is replaced by that of *stasis** (a term used by Dr. H. R. Carter, of the U.S. Public Health Service, a great authority on this disease, and the discoverer of the period of extrinsic incubation).

---

* "Yellow Fever, its Epidemiology, Prevention and Control." H. R. Carter. Supplement No. 19, U.S. Public Health Reports, 11th September, 1914.

The pains and distress disappear; the patient can now sleep or rests without sleeping. The appearance of the face changes, the active congestion of the skin and mucus membranes is replaced by passive congestion. "The face is no longer swollen, it is not bright red; shows a dusky pallor rather; the conjunctivæ are red, but with tortuous veins; they are dry rather than moist, making the dull-red eye of this stage. A distinct yellow colour is nearly always observable in the eyes."

"He lies flat in bed on his back; slides down on his pillow. The whole appearance of the man as he lies in bed is one of rest. His mind is clear; he speaks only when it is necessary to speak; speaks slowly, distinctly with a low voice; and he is tired, very, very tired."*

7. *Pyrexia.*—"Yellow Fever is not a disease of high temperatures. Rarely does it go over 103·5° F., even in bad cases. The temperature of light cases is highest on the first day. The temperature of moderate cases is highest on the first or second day and then commences to fall; 100° to 102·5° would include nine-tenths of all cases of Yellow Fever we get in this country (*i.e.*, America.) . . . . . The temperature goes on gradually down to the fourth or fifth day, or a little beyond the sixth day."*

8. *Albuminuria.*—The presence of albumen in the urine is, excluding Pyrexia, certainly the most constant symptom in Yellow Fever; it was only absent in a single case amongst those so classified by the Commission; in that case the evidence as to the nature of the disease was conclusive, both on clinical and on epidemiological grounds. (Case 23, Yellow Fever Report). It is not, however, the mere presence of albumen in the urine that is of so much importance, as that may happen in Malaria and other febrile disorders, but in Yellow Fever it appears with slight pyrexia, and is often out of proportion to the degree of fever. "When you find a man with a temperature of 101·5° to 102° with albumen that you have to shake out of the tube, that is not the ordinary albumen of high temperature of an ordinary infection."*

---

* Carter *Op. cit.*, p. 24.

It is usually found about the evening of the third day. "When it appears on the first day it goes to a fatal termination, on the second day it is of very bad augury."*

At first it is small in amount, but increases for the next two or three days, and may do so *whilst the temperature is falling and the quantity of urine is diminishing.*

It may persist until the sixth or eighth day and gradually disappear as the urine returns to the normal quantity. This correllated sequence of events does not occur, so far as we are aware, in any other disease for which Yellow Fever is likely to be mistaken. It was observed in all the less severe cases during the Lagos epidemic.

The finding of tube casts in the centrifugalised deposit, especially if bile stained, is valuable confirmatory evidence.

9. *High Temperature with a Slow Pulse.*—(Faget's sign). Unlike what usually happens in the majority of acute febrile disorders the pulse in Yellow Fever very often does not follow the rise and fall of the temperature. This is known as Faget's sign, and is undoubtedly often observed in Yellow Fever, but in the early period of the illness, when the difficulty of diagnosis is greatest, and the question most important, the pulse is often rapid, full and bounding. Moreover this condition is often met with in other diseases, but not often in Malaria. Faget's sign is sometimes present throughout, but usually appears later, during the remission of the fever, and the slow pulse rate may be prolonged into the stage of convalescence. Faget's sign was noted in 33 out of 38 cases in the Lagos epidemic of 1913.

It is not improbable that the slow pulse of Yellow Fever, and of other conditions in which jaundice is present, is to be attributed to a like cause.

10. *Condition of the Gums.*—The condition of the gums should be carefully noted in every case in which Yellow Fever is suspected, as it may give an important clue to the nature of the disease. They are very often red and swollen and later may bleed.

11. *The Tongue.*—The appearance of the tongue varies, as it does in every febrile disease, but the most typical condition is a

---

* H. R. Carter, *Op. cit.*, p. 26.

pointed tongue, with a white dorsum and red tip and edges. It is not uncommonly described as furred, with the tip and edges clean; later it becomes small, dry and brown.

12. *Nausea and vomiting.*—Nausea is rarely absent, vomiting more often so, particularly in the mild cases occurring amongst natives.

13. *Jaundice.*—It is often difficult in native adults, owing to the natural pigmentation of the sclerotics, to be sure of the presence of jaundice, although not so in native children. The time of appearance in 24 carefully observed cases, all of which recovered, in the Lagos epidemic of 1913, was as follows:—

Day of the disease.	Cases.
4th	3
5th	5
6th	5
7th	2
8th	2
9th	2
10th	1
11th	3
12th	1
	24

In all these cases the sclerae are mentioned as the first site in which the colouration was noticed.

14. *Skin rash.*—The occasional occurrence of a rash, which is generally described as erythematous, has often been observed in Yellow Fever.

The following are descriptions of such a condition in a European who recovered. On the 7th day of the illness it is noted:—

> "There was an erythematous blush on the skin of the back and chest. On the eighth the rash was more pronounced and rosy. It looked like the rash of measles and extended to the abdomen, arms and legs. It had not appeared on the face. The rash was accompanied by some pruritus."

In a fatal case in a European, on the 4th day of the illness it is noted that:—

> "A rash like measles appeared on the face, the upper part of the trunk and the backs of the hands. Two days later it was fading, and after a similar interval it had disappeared, to be replaced by petechiæ about the neck and trunk and on the hands."

In a European æt. 45, in whom the disease was fatal, it is noted that "the skin is yellowish-red, almost the colour of brawn."

In a rapidly fatal case in a European, on the 4th day "an erythematous rash appeared on the skin of the neck and chest."

In a similar case, also in a European, it is noted on the 3rd day that "the skin is covered with a red rash."

15. *Epigastric Pulsation.*—Special stress was laid by Dr. Paez (*vide* p. 162) on this symptom, which, so far as we are aware, has not hitherto been observed.

16. *Other symptoms.*—Brief mention may be made of the following symptoms, as their presence or absence should always be noted in doubtful cases:—

> Photophobia, thirst, a peculiar odour of the body described as "fishy," epistaxis, constipation, high coloured urine, pigmentation of the nails.

(*B*) DIAGNOSIS OF CASES OF THE SEVERE TYPE.

It would carry us far beyond the scope of this report to consider in detail the phenomena which may be met with in cases of Yellow Fever of the severe or hæmorrhagic type; moreover, it is unnecessary, as they are fully described in the text books, particularly those devoted to tropical diseases.

It may, however, be of service to comment briefly upon certain features which have been observed in cases which have come under the notice of the Commission.

Onset.—The onset of the illness in these, as in the milder cases, is usually sudden, and attended by rigor or sensations of chilliness, but a gradual onset is not uncommon, and does not preclude a severe or fatal attack. With what frequency "ambulant" cases occur amongst the natives is quite unknown.

In the Abeokuta case (*vide* p. 54) the patient had been feeling ill for three or four days before the onset of the serious symptoms, and was able to travel by rail to Lagos, yet the attack was fatal. A native who walked to the hospital stated that he had been ill for six days previously, yet the attack was severe. In the native cases it is not uncommon to find that they have been at work during the period of the disease to which it is believed the power of infecting a mosquito is limited. The following are examples of this:—

> "The patient states that he felt ill four days ago, with a sensation of chilliness and headache. He continued at his work for a couple of days, but felt worse each day."—Lagos, Case 24.
>
> "Patient states that he felt ill on the sixteenth, but continued at his work all that day. Next day, though still feeling 'seedy,' he went to work again, but that night he had a severe frontal headache. * * * * * *."—Lagos, Case 28.

On reference to the sporadic cases (p. 57) it will be seen that the patient from Ogbomosho was taken off a passenger train, not because he complained of illness, but owing to the fact that he was found to have a temperature of 103°F.

In a Syrian, who died of Yellow Fever, the history of the onset of his illness was as follows:—

> "On May 18th the patient complained of feeling tired and of yawning and stretching himself frequently. On May 19th all the above feelings were exaggerated. On May 20th he took a dose of Epsom salts, but the tiredness was not relieved thereby. He sought medical advice at 6 p.m, when the temperature was 101° F."—Case 8, Yellow Fever Report.

In the Second Report (p. 125) the details are given of a remarkable case of Yellow Fever in a European, in which for five days the symptoms justified the diagnosis of Catarrhal Jaundice; yet on the sixth day the temperature, which had hitherto been normal, suddenly rose to 101°F then to 106°F. The patient became comatose, albumen appeared in the urine, dark fluid came from the mouth, and death followed on the following day. The post-mortem appearances were typical of Yellow Fever.

The consideration of other signs and symptoms in the cases of the severe type is deferred to the following section on "Differential Diagnosis."

SECTION XI.

DIFFERENTIAL DIAGNOSIS.

(*A*) The Differential Diagnosis of Malaria and Yellow Fever.

As this enquiry has proceeded it has become obvious that the most debatable question is still, as it has always been, the differential diagnosis of Malaria and Yellow Fever.

The Second Report of the Commission contains many illustrations of the fact that in the past cases of Yellow Fever have been diagnosed as Malaria, but it is not likely that the opposite error has often been made. Everywhere throughout the world the influence of Governments and of local popular opinion has been against a recognition of the fact that Yellow Fever was within their borders. Terror of the disease and fear of the effect of the announcement upon trade have generally been the determining factors.

Those concerned took less trouble to learn to distinguish the one disease from the other, because they had determined beforehand, if possible, never to admit the existence of Yellow Fever.

Augustin gives a list of 152 names which have been at one period or another in use to describe the disease; indeed, the writers of all nationalities appear to have vied with each other in the production of names, many of them doubtless invented with the sole purpose of avoiding the use of the term "Yellow Fever" and implying that it is really a form of Malaria.

ond ɔort, 40.

As already stated, "the Commission are of opinion that the day has gone by for endeavouring by the use of euphemistic terms to conceal the presence of Yellow Fever, and that the only hope of eradicating the disease lies in boldly facing the facts."

ond ort, o.

Again, "It is to be particularly noted that with a change in the observer temporarily in charge, 'Yellow Fever' immediately appears in a place where 'bilious remittent fever,' 'bilious hæmaturic fever,' and 'malignant (hyperpyrexia) fever' had recently been present." One of the most comprehensive names, which is of frequent occurrence in the West African reports, is "bilious remittent hæmorrhagic fever."

When the symptoms of two diseases having a resemblance to one another are enumerated on paper without comment or explanation, it may appear to the inexperienced either impossible to mistake the one for the other, or impossible to differentiate them; nevertheless, almost a single glance may be sufficient to enable a practised clinician to decide with which of the two he is dealing. In the recognition of disease there is much that cannot be written down so clearly that he who reads may see, if it were not so a "Family

Encyclopædia of Medicine" would suffice for diagnosis. The vomiting of any black material may be "black vomit" to one who has never seen it in Yellow Fever, but it is not necessarily so to a physician experienced in the diagnosis of that disease.

Dr. Felix Paez, Chief of the Medical Department of the Hospital Ruiz, Ciudad Bolivar, Venezuela, who has had very considerable experience of Yellow Fever in that country, kindly attended a meeting of the Commission and gave interesting evidence on the question of the differential diagnosis of the bilious remittent type of Malaria from Yellow Fever and on other points.

The following is an *epitomé* of Dr. Paez' views:—

(1) He recognised three types of Yellow Fever:—

(i.) A very mild form=20 per cent.
(ii.) The common form=60 per cent.
(iii.) A severe form=20 per cent.

There was not much difficulty in differentiating Malaria from Yellow Fever. Bilious remittent fever was recognised as Malaria; it was characterised by vomiting and jaundice. Only very mild cases of Yellow Fever could be mistaken for bilious remittent. Including these mild cases, hæmorrhages from the nose or gums or elsewhere would be found in 95 per cent. (*sic*) of the cases of Yellow Fever, if carefully looked for. A peculiar sniffing or sighing type of breathing was frequently present in Yellow Fever.

(2) The pulse was high in Malaria, but low in Yellow Fever. He attached great importance to Faget's sign, which was absent in Malaria. He had seen a pulse of 38 in convalescence and 45 was common.

(3) He also attached importance to the appearance, increase, decline and disappearance of albumen in the urine; albuminuria was not present in Malaria of the bilious remittent type: to the lessened quantity of the urine and its high specific gravity.

(4) Also to the appearance of jaundice on the third day, rarely on the second; usually slight at first, but sometimes very intense. Some of the slight cases did not show any jaundice.

(5) Also to the facial appearance, but this was not absolutely diagnostic. Two or three definite signs must be assembled before a case could be recognised with certainty.

(6) He laid special stress upon epigastric pain and *pulsation*, the latter could be seen. It occurred in very mild cases of Yellow Fever. It was not, in his opinion, hepatic or due to over distension of the right side of the heart; probably it was derived from the cœliac artery. It was never present in Malaria.

(7) The vomit in the first instance was alimentary, then bilious and then would contain specks of blood, "fly specks" or red blood filaments. There might be a vomit of red blood, especially in children. Sometimes there would be a black vomit, like coffee, at other times only "fly specks."

(8) The liver and spleen were commonly enlarged in bilious remittent fever, whereas enlargement of the liver was rare in Yellow Fever, and the spleen was seldom or never enlarged in ordinary cases, but it might be so in very severe cases.

(9) The temperature in Malaria might drop quickly to the normal in one day. If a Yellow Fever patient also suffered from a malarial paroxysm the typical remission on the third day would not be observed. He did not think that *latent* Malaria would modify the course of Yellow Fever.

(10) Fever of the bilious remittent type was, in his opinion, more common as the earliest, than as a subsequent, manifestation of Malaria.

(11) He had seen death from Malaria. Consciousness was lost and the heart failed, whereas in Yellow Fever they died of anuria, sometimes with convulsions.

(12) He had seen hyperpyrexial fever, it was really pernicious Malaria.

The Commission are indebted to Dr. Felix Paez for the translation from "Yellow Fever, by Dr. Luis Cuervo Marquiz" of the following tabular statement with comments on the differential diagnosis of Yellow Fever and Bilious Remittent Malarial Fever :—

"DIFFERENTIAL DIAGNOSIS OF YELLOW FEVER FROM BILIOUS REMITTENT MALARIAL FEVER.

"*Bilious Remittent Fever.*	*Yellow Fever.*
"(1). It is localised to intense marshy foci.	(1) It is observed in places where malaria does not exist and is absent in others intensely paludic.
"(2). It is found particularly in the open country.	(2). Particularly found in towns or where there are collections of people.
"(3). It spares new comers, and it is usually preceded by advanced malarial conditions.	(3). New comers are most frequently attacked. It is not preceded by malarial conditions.
"(4). The first attack predisposes to others.	(4). A first attack preserves from further ones.
"(5). It is not transmissible.	(5). It is transmissible.
"(6). It is sporadic, or may affect the epidemic form after great floods, and at the beginning or end of the rainy season.	(6). It is epidemic or endemo-epidemic. The influence of floods has not been well established.
"(7). There are generally prodromal symptoms.	(7). The invasion is generally sudden.
"(8). During the period of invasion the face does not present any noticeable feature.	(8). The *facial syndrome*, characterised by the turgescence of the skin of the face, the congestion of the ocular and buccal mucosæ, and more particularly of the palatine and gingival mucosæ, is typical of yellow fever, and is comparable only with those of eruptive fevers. It is not constant in the mild form.
"(9). The skin does not present any characteristic feature. It is pale, moist, without patches or rashes during the invasion. Ecchymoses and large blood effusions of the cellular tissue are exceptional.	(9). The skin is congested at the initial period and turns yellow during the second and third. These hæmorrhages are not present as a general rule, but are met with frequently.
"(10). Hæmorrhages are present in a restricted number of cases. Epistaxis as a rule is very slight. Hæmatemesis, enterorhægia and other hæmorrhages of mucosæ are so rare that some authors, as Dutraulau and Vallin, deny their existence. "Hæmorrhages cannot be considered as symptoms of remittent fever, but as complications.	(10). Hæmorrhages are constant symptoms. In the mild form they may be confined to slight epistaxis or be totally absent.
"(11). The temperature rises and maintains during the stadium period for some time with morning remissions and evening rises. The oscillations may be of 1·5°, 2°, 2·5°, between morning and evening temperatures.	(11). The temperature rises rapidly during the first 12 or 36 hours to the maximum. Then a remission may follow, which in many cases may go on to a complete defervescence or it may rise again to the initial figure, to go down again in a rapid or oscillating manner.
"(12). The recurrences during remission, which are only the continuation of the fever, are the rule.	(12). Recurrence is rare. The period of calm is constant.
"(13) Jaundice is an early symptom.	(13). Jaundice is relatively late.
"(14). There is no diminution in the quantity of urine nor anuria, except when there is some renal complication. Albuminuria may be present in grave cases. The urine is bilious.	(14). Albuminuria and the diminution of the quantity of urine which may go on to anuria are constant in grave cases. The urine seldom contains bile.

" *Bilious Remittent Fever.*	*Yellow Fever.*
" (15). Cephalalgia and rachialgia are moderate. The first is seldom localized.	(15). Cephalalgia and rachiulgia are constant and intense. Cephalalgia is localized in the frontal region.
" (16). Meningo-encephalic manifestations are of no importance and are frequently absent.	(16). Meningo-encephalic conditions are constant.
" (17). Indefinite duration.	(17). The evolution lasts a week or a week and a half.
" (18). Convalescence is slow and there is weakness. Malarial manifestations may follow.	(18). Convalescence is easy.
" (19). Nothing particular occurs during convalescence.	(19). Depression, hypothermia and slowness of the pulse are nearly constant.
" (20). Quinine is the remedy for the disease.	(20). Quinine fails.
" (21). Post-mortem shows infections of the spleen and liver, and black dots on the surface of the brain, especially in the bulb.	(21). The liver is either enlarged, or normal or small and generally yellow. The spleen is normal or small, except when there is a malarial condition co-existing.
" (22). The fever is frequently followed by intermittent fits.	(22). Intermittent fits are met with only when there is existing malaria.
" (23). The mortality is great, but not to the proportions of yellow fever. Generally, death is the consequence of a series of attacks.	(23). There is a higher mortality than in the remittent fever.

" The diagnosis is a very easy one to be made theoretically, as we see, but in practice there are cases in which the most experienced practitioner is doubtful about the disease he has to confront.

" In a remittent fever cephalalgia, severe rachialgia, nausea and vomiting, albuminuria, epistaxis, jaundice, that is to say, the syndrome of a case of yellow fever of medium intensity, may be met.

" Similarly, in a case of yellow fever one may find cephalalgia, moderate rachialgia, bilious vomits, slight remittence, early jaundice, bilious urine and the whole aspect of the remittent fever. In these cases it is very difficult to make a diagnosis when yellow fever and remittent fever co-exist in the same place.

" In our opinion, to settle the matter from the first moment is impossible, and that only by a close and attentive examination of the preceding conditions, of the progress of the disease, by a grouping of the symptoms rather than by isolated symptoms, we may obtain the elements to make a diagnosis which will be always of a reserved character. And still there are cases in which even *a posteriori* one cannot say which disease one has dealt with.

" Putting aside the etiological elements, which sometimes are conclusive, we think that in the first stage the *facial syndrome;* in the second stage the thermie remission, the albuminuria, the jaundice, the slowness of the pulse; in the third stage the multiple hæmorrhages, the diminution or suppression of urine and the aspect of the vomit; in the convalescence the hypothermia, the depression, the slowness of the pulse, and in the whole course of the disease a particular aspect of the patient, which you see but which you cannot describe, are the salient features which practically separate the two diseases."

It will be noticed that on some points the views of Dr. Cuervo Marquiz and Dr. Paez are not in accord.

Dr. Paez is of opinion that the bilious remittent type of Malaria can only simulate the very mild type of Yellow Fever, whereas it is clear from the tabular statement of Dr. Marquiz that it may resemble the more severe type.

Again, fever of the bilious remittent type, in Dr. Paez' opinion, is more common as the earliest than as a subsequent manifestation of Malaria, whereas Dr. Marquiz considers that it is usually preceded by advanced malarial conditions.

It is clear from the omission of any mention of the possible presence of parasites and pigmented leucocytes in the blood in Malaria, and their absence in uncomplicated Yellow Fever, that at the date at which Dr. Marquiz wrote this aid to diagnosis had not been discovered.

Dr. G. C. Low in a paper on the "Differential Diagnosis of Yellow Fever and Malignant Malaria" (B.M.J., September 20th, 1902, p. 860) reviews the various symptoms of the two diseases and concludes thus:—

> "It is fortunate, with all these symptoms in so many ways resembling each other, that we possess an almost decisive method of at once determining between the two diseases—namely, the examination of the blood for the malarial parasites.
>
> "It is true that in some cases the parasites of malignant malaria may be extremely scanty in the peripheral blood, and repeated search may be necessary to find them; but, as a rule, this does not hold good, one or two glances through the microscope often being sufficient to clear up the matter, parasites and corroborative evidence in the shape of pigmented leucocytes being seen. Of course, quinine must not have been administered before the examination of the blood is made; if this drug has been recently given a negative result is of no value."

It has been calculated upon the basis of certain standards, which it is unnecessary to set out in detail here, that the lowest number of parasites in the body capable of producing a first attack of Malarial Fever is:—

> "At least one parasite to 100.000 hæmatids; that is, 50 parasites in 1 c.mm. of blood; or 150,000,000 in a man of 10 stone (64 kilograms) in weight."

"The Prev[ention] of Malaria," [R.] Ross, 1910 pp. 90-94.

Also that:—

> " If the parasites are so few as this we can expect to find them at the rate of about one every quarter of an hour. But chance intervenes here: if we are lucky we may find the first parasite almost at once; if we are unlucky we may have to search several hundreds of thousands of hæmatids before finding an infected one. There is always the danger of overlooking a plasmodium when it should have been seen."
>
> " In the thick-film process (1903) 1 c.mm. of blood occupies only about one-fifth of a square c.m. of area or less, so that there should be twenty to thirty times more hæmatids and parasites per field."
>
> " Such calculations demonstrate the absurdity of supposing that there are no plasmodia present in a person because we fail in finding one after a few minutes' search. As a matter of fact, even if as many as 150,000,000 plasmodia are present in an average man, the chances are that ten to fifteen minutes' search will be required for each plasmodium found; while if we are careless or unfortunate we may have to look much longer."

If therefore the fever is due to Malaria, and the observer is competent, and his search sufficiently prolonged, the parasites should be found.

The consideration of this question of diagnosis is continued in the following sections on "Albuminuria in Malaria" and on "The Diagnostic Significance of the Presence of Malaria Parasites in cases of Pyrexia and on their absence."

Quite recently a paper has appeared in the American "Journal of Tropical Diseases and Preventive Medicine" on "A method of Concentrating Malaria Plasmodia for Diagnostic and Other Purposes," by C. C. Bass, M.D., and F. M. Johns, M.D., of the Tulane College of Medicine, New Orleans (p. 298-303), which may possibly prove of very great assistance in the differential diagnosis of Malaria and Yellow Fever.

The paper commences as follows:—

> " While working in Panama upon the cultivation of Malaria plasmodia during the summer of 1912, we discovered that whenever defibrinated or citrated blood containing crescents was centrifuged at a high rate of speed for a sufficient length of time these plasmodia rose to the top of the cell column, and that by this means a mass of almost pure crescents could be obtained from blood containing large numbers of them. The possibilities of this method of concentration of plasmodia for diagnostic and other purposes were at once appreciated after we had learned by further experiment that both the gametes and the schizonts of the other species of plasmodia could be concentrated in the same way."

The principles involved are thus explained:—

"The fundamental principles involved are the fact that a malaria plasmodium with its host erythrocyte is larger than the non-parasitized erythrocytes, and that when centrifuged at proper speed for sufficient length of time the larger cells rise to the top of the cell column, while the smaller cells collect beneath. Most of the leucocytes are still larger than most of the parasitized cells and accordingly rise to a higher level in the cell column, in fact, to the surface. After sufficient centrifuging, we have in the tube from the bottom upward, non-parasitized erythrocytes, parasitized erythrocytes, leucocytes and serum. If citrated, in place of defibrinated, blood is centrifuged, a greater or less amount of platelets settles upon the leucocyte layer, but unless it is centrifuged for a long time at high speed, most of them remain suspended in the supernatant plasma. The older and larger the parasites, the more certainly and promptly do they collect at the top when the blood is centrifuged. Crescents, other mature gametes, and tertian and quartan schizonts more than half grown, rise much more quickly than smaller parasites. In fact, many of the very smallest rings of the æstivo-autumnal species do not rise at all and little concentration of these can be obtained. The large ring forms and ameboid parasites of all species rise promptly. By proper technique ninety per cent. or more of all the plasmodia (except the smallest rings in which the percentage is considerably lower) can be collected from 10 cc. of blood and all placed upon one or two slides in the form of ordinary blood spreads. Of course, in very heavy infections, the total quantity of plasmodia may be too great for it all to be made into one or two ordinary blood spreads."

"The Ross thick film method, with which almost all workers on malaria are familiar, increases the chances of finding plasmodia in a search of a given length of time approximately ten times, since it is possible to examine in this way a film as much as ten times thicker than the thickest ordinary blood film that can be satisfactorily examined. The method has the advantage of being adaptable to field work, while our method would be applicable for diagnostic purposes to office and hospital work and only to a somewhat limited extent to general field work.

Assuming that one cc. of blood would make about one hundred ordinary blood spreads, and that at least 90 per cent. of all the plasmodia (except small æstivo-autumnal rings) present in 10 cc. of blood, can be collected and placed on one spread, the advantage over the ordinary blood spread method appears to be approximately 900 times. In other words, one minute spent in looking for plasmodia in a specimen prepared by this method should yield the same results as 900 minutes, or 15 hours, spent examining an ordinary blood spread. There is no reason why the idea of the Ross thick film method should not be combined with our method if desired, which would increase the efficiency to 9,000 times the ordinary blood spread method."

The description of the complete technique is too long for reproduction here and the reader is referred to the original paper.

The plates which accompany the paper give a very good idea of the degree of concentration which can be obtained by this method.

The long period which the authors have devoted to the perfection of the technique before publishing their results is a useful example to all workers in science, and increases the probability that the method will come into general use and will prove of great value in the differential diagnosis of Malaria and Yellow Fever.

(*B*) Albuminuria in Malaria and Yellow Fever.

The Commission have devoted considerable attention to the subject of the occurrence of albuminuria in Malaria, and have received much assistance from the work of the Investigators and from the evidence of witnesses who have kindly given them the benefit of their experience.

The question is one of great importance, in view of the contention that albuminuria is of such frequent occurrence in Malaria, that in the differentiation of that disease from Yellow Fever its presence in any case of suspected Yellow Fever is of little diagnostic value.

The statements in the text books and in the literature of the subject indicate considerable divergence of view, some authors being of opinion that this association is of frequent occurrence, whilst by others it is regarded as extremely rare.

ropical eases," Edition, 4, p. 55.

Sir Patrick Manson writes as follows:—

> "*The Urine in Ague.*—During the cold stage the urine is often limpid and abundant, and is passed frequently; but during the hot and sweating stages it is scanty, loaded, sometimes albuminous."

Subsequently the same author, in describing the clinical forms of Malarial Fevers, observes:—

l, p. 71.

> "It is neither necessary nor desirable to attempt to describe in detail the infinite variety malarial attacks exhibit. It would be impossible in a limited space to do so; and if done the result would amount only to an uninteresting and unprofitable ringing of the changes on rigor, pyrexia, diaphoresis, bilious vomiting, bilious diarrhœa, constipation, catarrhal gastritis, headache, boneache, prostration and so forth."

It is of interest to note that in this list of symptoms neither albuminuria nor any more severe renal complication is mentioned.

We shall therefore probably not be misrepresenting Sir Patrick Manson's views in concluding that in his experience albuminuria is not a common complication of Malaria.

Sir Leonard Rogers states:—

"*The Urine in Malaria.*

"The urine may be increased during the cold stage and decreased and of high specific gravity after the sweating one, but it very rarely shows albumen or other marked changes in uncomplicated cases."

"Fevers in the Tropics 2nd Edition p. 207.

The same author, under "The Urine in Yellow Fever," states:—

"Of still greater importance is the presence of ALBUMEN (*sic*), as the prognosis largely depends on the quantity present; moreover, it has considerable diagnostic value. The date of its appearance is very variable, although it rarely appears on the first day (3 per cent.), becomes more common on the second day (18 per cent.), and is most usually first evident on the third and fourth (55 per cent.), appearing with diminishing frequency after the fifth day. It varies from a trace up to an amount sufficient to completely solidify the fluid on boiling. The quantity of urea excreted in the twenty-four hours is also reduced in yellow fever, and very markedly so in many of the more severe attacks, much in proportion to their severity. Granular and hyaline casts may be present at any period, and blood corpuscles and detrities in addition in the second stage."

Ibid, p. 27

The same author, in discussing the diagnosis of Yellow Fever, writes as follows:—

"Such mild cases are most likely to be mistaken for a malignant tertian malaria, especially if complicated by the hæmoglobinuria of blackwater fever, the temperature curves being not at all dissimilar. The microscope is the surest means of differentiating between them, for the finding of malarial parasites, or in blackwater fever an increase and pigmentation of the large mononuclears, will enable those diseases to be recognised. The pulse is also a very important guide, for it is nearly always rapid during the pyrexia of malarial fever, but soon becomes slowed down in yellow fever.

Ibid, p. 27

"Relapsing fever is said also to be easily mistaken for yellow fever * * * * * * in both the above diseases albumen is rarely found in the urine, except during hæmoglobinuria complication, whilst it is present in yellow fever after the second day."

It is clear from the above statements that the author does not regard albuminuria as other than a rare complication of Malaria.

Castellani and Chalmers (2nd Edition, p. 863) under "Malaria," state:—

"During the attack the urine is at first increased in quantity. * * * * * *. Notwithstanding this increase in quantity the specific gravity is raised * * * * * * the colour is dark and the acidity of the urine is increased * * * * * *. Serum-albumen may be present after severe attacks, and proteose has been reported, as well as nucleoproteid. When the intermission comes, the urine diminishes in quantity * * * * * *. During convalescence the most marked features are the polyuria with low specific gravity, which in subtertian fevers may be so marked as to alarm the patient * * * * * *."

The same authors (p. 883) under "(*b*) Pernicious Fevers with Local Symptoms":—

"*Comatose Pernicious Fever.*—The urine, which may have casts and a little albumen, is usually passed involuntarily, as are the motions."

These authors are also clearly of opinion that albuminuria is only a rare complication of Malaria, and that it is, as a rule, only met with in severe attacks of that disease, in which other unmistakable symptoms are present.

1, p. 417, 7. Dr. Charles F. Craig, in the article on the Malarial Fevers in Osler and McCrae's "System of Medicine," writes as follows:—

"TERTIAN AND QUARTAN MALARIA.

"*The Cold Stage.*

"* * * * * * *. The urine is increased in quantity and lowered in specific gravity."

"During the cold stage an excessive amount of urine is often voided, polyuria being a most frequent symptom."

"Albuminuria is present in a considerable proportion of cases. Of over 1,000 cases of tertian infection, personally observed, nearly 400 showed albumen in the urine and 86 showed the presence of a few granular and epithelial casts." (p. 418.)

"SYMPTOMS OF TERTIAN ÆSTIVO-AUTUMNAL FEVER.

"*Hot Stage.*

"The urine is increased in quantity and is generally albuminous."

This is evidence that, in America, during a malarial attack, presenting a typical cold and hot stage, and therefore easily recognisable by those and other features, albumen may be found in the urine in a considerable percentage of cases.

7, 428, 429. The same author, under "Complications and Sequelæ," states:—

"The most common disease of the *genito-urinary* system complicating malaria is nephritis. Some form of nephritis occurred in at least 4 per cent. of æstivo-autumnal infections and in about ½ per cent. of tertian infections personally observed.

"It is more frequently a sequela of malaria than a complication."

Also, later (p. 431), under "Sequelæ of Malaria":—

"Among diseases of the genito-urinary system albuminuria is of frequent occurrence during acute attacks of malaria, and oftentimes persists for some time after the cessation of such attacks. Thayer and Hewetson found albuminuria in over 50 per cent. of their cases. Thayer found that it was most frequent in æstivo-autumnal infections, occurring in 58·3 per cent. of these infections, in contrast to 38·6 per cent. of tertian and quartan infections. Rem-Pici has contributed most extensively to our knowledge of the albuminurias occurring during and after malarial infections. From personal experience albuminuria occurs in about 50 per cent. of cases of æstivo-autumnal and in about 30 to 35 per cent. of cases of tertian and quartan malaria.

"Both acute and chronic nephritis may occur as sequelæ of the malarial fevers. * * * * * *. Personal observations suggest that nephritis occurs in at least 3 per cent. of all cases of æstivo-autumnal infections, the most common form being chronic parenchymatous. It is rare in tertian and quartan infections, but is always found in fatal cases."

A "complication" of a disease is an event of occasional occurrence during the course of the disease, certainly not one of its distinctive features. Similarly, a "sequela" of a disease is a lesion sometimes met with after the acute symptoms distinctive of the disease have disappeared.

Applying these tests to the occurrence of albuminuria in Yellow Fever and Malaria respectively we observe that in the former disease it is invariably present, appears at or about a certain day, continues for a variable period, and, in cases which recover, disappears as the illness passes off, without leaving permanent effects upon the renal organs; whereas in the hospital cases of Malaria at Baltimore, upon which these observations were made, presumably severe cases, nephritis was found more frequently as a sequela than as a complication, but in only 3 per cent. of such infections. The small amount of albumen found in the large proportion—50 per cent. to 38 per cent.—of the cases observed at Baltimore is mentioned in the extracts from Dr. Thayer's article on "Malaria" in Allbutt and Rolleston's "System of Medicine," quoted below.

The paper by Thayer and Hewetson referred to above in Dr. Craig's article is based on the records of 616 cases of Malarial Fever treated in the wards and out-patient department of the Johns Hopkins Hospital between the years 1889 and 1894.

Thayer & Hewetson. "The Malarial Fevers of Baltimore." Johns Hopk. Hosp. Rep. 1896, Vol. p. 5.

It is of interest to note, as reference is made to the statement in a later section of this report (*vide* p. 183) that "excepting two or three instances where the patients entered the hospital during convalescence, the specific micro-organism was found in every case of Malarial Fever treated in the wards."

The condition of the urine is thus described (p. 73):—

"*Urine.*—The analysis of the urine in the 335 cases occurring in the hospital shows the following results:—

"The urine was normal in 151 instances.

"Albumen was noted in 133 instances.

"Casts of the renal tubes were found in 31 instances.

"The 'diazo' reaction was present in 18 instances.

"Acute hæmorrhagic nephritis was present in 3 instances.

"Severe subacute diffuse nephritis was present in 1 instance.

"No note was made in 51 instances.

"In not a single instance of malarial fever observed in the hospital or in the out-patient department was hæmaturia present, with the exception of the three cases of acute nephritis, where the blood was present in the shape of altered red corpuscles, giving a smoky character to the urine."

Dr. Thayer in the article on "Malaria" in Allbutt and Rolleston's "System of Medicine" makes a fuller statement as to the amount of albumen found in the Johns Hopkins Hospital cases:—

II., "*The Urine in Malaria.*—* * * * * *. In the regularly inter-
II., mittent fevers, tertian and quartan, a trace of albumen was present
3. in 38·6 per cent. of 352 cases in the wards of the Johns Hopkins Hospital. In æstivo-autumnal fever it was more frequent, occurring in 58·3 per cent. of 165 cases. In the great majority of instances there was only a slight trace. In many of the cases in which albumen is found occasional hyaline casts may be detected in the sediment. In pernicious fever traces of bile may be found."

And later in the same article the following occurs (p. 365):—

"*Nephritis.*—Acute nephritis is not an uncommon sequel, occurring in 1·7 per cent. of 1,832 cases analysed at the Johns Hopkins Hospital. Rare in tertian and quartan infections, it is by no means infrequent in æstivo-autumnal fever. There is nothing remarkable in the character of the disease, which pursues the course of an ordinary acute toxic nephritis. Of 26 cases of malarial nephritis 14 recovered; 4 died; in 9 the result was doubtful; in 2 chronic nephritis followed. We have since seen several additional cases of chronic nephritis of undoubted malarial origin."

. Thayer, The same author in "Lectures on the Malarial Fevers"
31. states:—

"*Albumen.*—Albumen is usually present after severe paroxysms. In the regularly intermittent fevers it may amount only to a slight trace, whilst in severe infections it may be more abundant.

"The *sediment* here shows usually a few hyaline or granular casts. In the milder cases these are *only to be found after the most prolonged and careful search.* Where the albumen is more abundant they may be frequent. Italics not the origina

"Acute nephritis occasionally occurs in connection with or following malarial infection. Here the sediment shows numerous hyaline, granular and epithelial casts, and in some instances blood.

"Malarial fever may be followed by severe chronic nephritis; here the quantity of albumen may be abundant (one half per cent. or more), while the sediment may show numerous casts and renal epithelial cells."

Osler (7th Edition, p. 15) states under "Morbid Anatomy":—

"3. The accidental and late associations of malarial fever:—

"(*c*) *Nephritis.*—Moderate albuminuria is a frequent occurrence, having occurred in 46·4 per cent. of the cases in my wards. Acute nephritis is relatively frequent in æstivo-autumnal infections, having occurred in over 4·5 per cent. of my cases. Chronic nephritis occasionally follows long continued or frequently repeated infections."

Dr. David G. Willets, in an article on "Malaria in the Philippine General Hospital, Manila, P.I., during the fiscal year, 1913," gives under "Miscellaneous Hospital Findings":—

"The Philippine Journal of Science," IX., Sec. No. 5, September, 19 p. 445.

"TABLE III.--URINALYSIS.*

	Number.	Per cent.
Persons not examined	28	—
Persons examined	157	—
Persons negative	3	1·9
Persons with—		
Albumen	73	46·5
Albumen and casts	38	24·2
Albumen casts, pus cells and red cells	13	8·3
Albumen and pus cells	9	5·7
Albumen and red cells	8	5·1
Albumen casts and red cells ...	8	5 1
Albumen casts and pus cells ...	3	1·9
Albumen pus cells and red cells ...	2	1·3
	157	100·0

* *Author's Note.*—"As a rule but one morning specimen of urine was examined. The heat and acetic acid test was used for albumen."

We shall now proceed to consider the evidence bearing on this question contained in the reports from Investigators and the evidence of witnesses, many of whom were able to speak as to the condition of the urine in Malaria, as that disease is observed amongst Europeans and natives on the West Coast of Africa.

Lt.-Colonel Statham, who investigated on behalf of the Commission at Sierra Leone a series of 800 cases of medical pyrexia in 1913, and whose report thereon, and also on a further series of 300 cases of the same nature of earlier date, is contained in the Second Volume of Investigators' Reports (pp. 353-386) states (p. 359):—

> "Of 150 urine examinations which time has permitted me to look up, half in Europeans and half in natives, albumen was present in 9 of 75 cases amongst the former and 32 of 75 amongst the latter.
>
> "The presence of traces of albumen in natives is largely due, I believe, to urethral affections. Possibly ankylostomiasis, so prevalent among them, may also account for the presence of albumen in their urine. Casts were rarely or never found in these native albuminurias."

We have analysed Table IV. (p. 364) of Colonel Statham's Report, which deals with 71 cases of fever of a doubtful nature amongst adults, with the following results:—

(1) Malarial parasites were not found in any of the 71 cases, but it is noted in many of the cases that quinine had been given.

(2) Of 39 cases in which there is a record of the condition of the urine as regards albumen it was absent in 38, of which 17 are regarded as Malaria, either on clinical grounds or from the effect of quinine.

(3) Many of the cases in which the condition of the urine is not noted were also regarded as cases of Malaria.

(4) A slight cloud of albumen was present *in only one case* (No 71), which is classed as "?Typhus, Dengue type, 3 distinct rashes."

It does not therefore appear that albuminuria is of frequent occurrence in cases of pyrexia of a doubtful nature amongst adults at Sierra Leone whether Europeans, West Indians or natives.

Dr. G. G. Butler, in a Report on work carried out at Sierra Leone in 1913, also contained in the Second Volume of Investigators'

Reports (pp. 389 to 416), p. 397' deals with this qestion as follows:—

"The presence of albumen has been the point to which particular attention has been directed. Amongst the in-patients a difficulty has been met with owing to the untrustworthiness of the native dressers, *e.g.*, one specimen of urine was watered down and made to serve as specimens from four different patients."

"The question of small quantities of albumen in the urine has appeared to me to be an important point to investigate, on the supposition that a mild case of yellow fever may well show only a trace of albumen, for I have assumed that the less toxic the condition of the patient the less likelihood is there of any damage to the kidneys, or, in other words, that the albuminuria may be a measure of the severity of the illness."

Dr. Butler examined as a control 437 urines from hospital out-patients, irrespective of their illness, of these in 248 albumen was absent; in 189, *i.e.*, 43 per cent. albumen was present, in quantity from a trace upwards. Of these it was present in "some quantity" in 60 cases:—

"These figures only give a rough idea of the prevalence of slight cases of albuminuria in patients examined in a routine fashion and quite irrespective of their illnesses.

"The cause of their condition appears to be largely the prevalence of chronic urethral disease; among the Freetown natives of the hospital class a prostatitis or gleet is almost the rule above a certain age, and the presence of prostatic threads with the absence of casts is suggestive that the albumen is not of kidney origin.

"Owing to this state of affairs the difficulty of associating the presence of albuminuria with the illness of the patients is unfortunately increased.

"Under the heading of malaria a statistical account will be given of the extent of albuminuria found associated with the condition—*without the elimination of urethral disease, however.*" (p. 398.)

Dr. Butler's results from the examination of the urine in the malarial cases were as follows (p. 403):—

"*Albuminuria.*—Urine examinations in these malarial cases has not been so frequent as I could wish: this has been due to two reasons—firstly, because the diagnosis of malaria having been made on the blood condition, before I had been put on my guard by the control observation, any further examination of the patient was supposed to be unnecessary; and secondly, because most of the malarial cases were out-patient cases which made this further procedure rather awkward. However, there have been 42 examinations of urine among the in-patient cases; 21 showed no albuminuria, and the remaining 21 showed its presence as a 'thin cloud' with the acidifying and boiling test. In one case there was quite a heavy cloud of albumen."

It will, however, be remembered that Dr. Butler found albumen in the urine in 43 per cent. of his control cases; if therefore we apply that experience to these 42 malaria cases it is obvious that the share taken by the malarial infection in the production of the albuminuria in the in-patient cases was either insignificant or, having regard to the fact that the figures only give "a rough idea" of the frequency of slight albuminuria, and also to the statement as to the untrustworthiness of the native dressers, that it had no effect whatever.

It is clear from the foregoing statement that it is necessary to be *extremely* careful in drawing conclusions as to the significance of albuminuria in natives, either that:—

(1) Malaria is commonly associated with albuminuria; or

(2) That a given case is possibly one of mild Yellow Fever as albumen is present in the urine; or

(3) That the mere presence of albumen in the urine in such patients has necessarily any significance, either as regards Malaria or Yellow Fever.

As already stated, more than once, it is not the presence of albumen in the urine which is the point of so much importance in the diagnosis of the mild type of Yellow Fever, but its appearance on or about a certain day, its increase, and its gradual disappearance during convalescence, accompanied by characteristic changes in the quantity of the urine.

Dr. G. E. H. Le Fanu has reported the results of an investigation of cases of fever at Quittah from March to June, 1914.

The cases numbered 106, of which 81 were in children, and 25 in adults from 17 years upwards.

The following diseases were met with:—

Malaria	94	(worm infections in 11)
Yellow Fever	3	
Helminthiasis	4	
? Enteritis	1	
Typhoid Fever	2	(1 doubtful)
Pulmonary Congestion ...	1	
Undiagnosed	1	
	106	

Malarial parasites were found in 88 of the cases diagnosed as Malaria, as follows:—

Subtertian	55
Tertian	19
Quartan	2
Subtertian and Tertian	4
Tertian and Quartan	2
Quartan and plasmodium tenue	1
Species not determined	5
	88

The following statement as regards the cases of Yellow Fever occurs in the Report:—

> "Three cases of yellow fever were observed. In one (No. 26), which was fatal, there could be no doubt as to the diagnosis In the second (Case 63) there seems to have been a latent malarial infection, as careful examination of the thick films repeatedly revealed the presence of pigment, though no parasites were found until the 8th day. The third case (No. 98) was slight and of short duration."

Table 1 of the Report contains a list of cases with albuminuria and jaundice.

Thirty-seven cases are included in this table, from which it appears that albuminuria was present in 34 cases:—

Slight	23
Marked	6
Very marked	5
Not examined	1
Absent	2
	37

Of the 37 cases included in this table, evidence of malarial infection was present in 28 cases.

Jaundice was observed in nine cases and worms were found in 15 cases.

Analysis of the table shows that the number of cases in children in which albuminuria was present is very large, viz., 20 out of 22, in one the urine was not examined and in one only was albumen absent. All these were cases of Malaria except one.

In eight cases in children aged 2 years and under, albumen was found in the urine; one of these was only 8 months old.

The nature of the test for albumen employed in these cases is not stated in the Report.

The following are all the statements of witnesses which have a bearing upon the question under discussion.

Sir Charles Pardey Lukis, K.C.S.I., Director-General of the Indian Medical Service, who kindly attended a meeting of the Commission, stated that a parenchymatous nephritis was common in Malaria in India.

Lt.-Colonel Statham stated to the Commission that albuminuria had been shown in only two or three out of some thirty cases of Malaria in Europeans, but in about one-third of the native cases.

Colonel Gorgas stated that albuminuria was very common in severe Malaria, and that the albuminuria in Malaria was more marked in negroes than in whites and subsided with the fever. In Yellow Fever there was a progressive decrease of the urine and increase of the albumen.

Dr. W. E. Deeks, chief of the medical clinic of the Ancon Hospital, Panama, who kindly gave evidence before the Commission, stated that in his experience albuminuria was present in almost *all severe cases of æstivo-autumnal Malaria.* It nearly always cleared up rapidly, and was simply a slight febrile albuminuria. Casts were also found. He was of opinion that in 80 per cent. of the cases of Malaria that he had seen albumen could be found by the cold nitric acid test, if the urine was examined when it was quite fresh. He had frequently seen 25 per cent. by bulk of albumen in the urine of such cases. There was no difficulty in distinguishing between cases of this kind and Yellow Fever, if the microscope was used. If a case of Malaria was untreated parasites could always be found. He had only seen about 20 cases of Yellow Fever.

Dr. Bailey stated at an interview that "since the occurrence of certain cases at Burutu and Forcados in 1913, 30 of which in natives he thought might be Yellow Fever, they had carried out from 200 to 300 tests of urine as they had applied the test to every one who said he had a headache. The albuminuria in these cases usually cleared up rapidly, and was obviously connected with the course of the fever. He had once found albuminuria in a European case of

Malaria, in which he had also found the parasite, but it was a mere trace, quite unlike this group of cases."

The late Dr. Mackinnon stated that "he used formerly to examine the urine in Malaria cases. He had not found much albuminuria."

Dr. Hutton stated that "he had not examined the urine to any considerable extent, as people were suspicious, and it was difficult to get specimens. In the case of the school children at Abokobi the specimens obtained showed no albumen."

At that school several children were found to have pyrexia due to malarial infection. One child had a temperature of 104° F., but was not inconvenienced by it.

Dr. E. W. Graham stated that "the results of examining the urine in Malaria cases had been negative as regards the presence of albumen."

Dr. Leonard informed the Commission that "he had not observed albuminuria in uncomplicated cases of Malaria. Whilst in charge of the native hospital at Calabar the urine was regularly examined. He had seen no albumen in cases of fever at Calabar, nor any cases resembling those diagnosed as Yellow Fever at Lagos."

Dr. Leonard also stated that "As to the occurrence of gleet, with as a result the presence of albumen in the urine, he had experienced no difficulty; as he found that in such cases if the patient passed urine, and then shortly afterwards a fresh specimen was collected and tested, there was, as a rule, no reaction. When there was, it was a slight one and there was nothing like the amount of albumen present in the Yellow Fever cases."

Dr. Hänschell stated that "every case admitted into the European or native hospital (at Sekondi) was tested for albuminuria. He supposed that he had tested nearly 300 in all. He had only found four cases in which albuminuria and Malaria were combined. There was albuminuria in 30 or 40 cases, but those patients were mostly there for surgical complaints, and many had had gonorrhœa recently or still had it. Others were cases of Pneumonia, and in three schistosome ova were found in the urine."

We are now in a position to formulate the conclusions which may be deduced from the evidence brought forward both generally and as regards West Africa.

Conclusions.

(1) There is evidence that in severe attacks of æstivo-autumnal Malaria accompanied by pyrexia, albumen may be present in the urine.

(2) That in such cases the amount of albumen is generally a mere trace.

(3) That the albuminuria does not run a clinical course in any way similar to that observed in Yellow Fever.

(4) That it is probably a pyrexial albuminuria, and is similar to that occasionally met with in Pneumonia, Typhoid Fever, and other acute febrile diseases.

(5) That casts may be present, but are only found in very severe cases of malarial pyrexia, whereas they are commonly met with in Yellow Fever, and may, in that disease, be bile stained.

(6) That the evidence from West Africa affords no support to the contention that albuminuria is of common occurrence in Malaria as observed in that country amongst Europeans.

(7) That the frequent occurrence of urethritis, either acute or chronic, amongst the natives of West Africa, indicates the necessity for eliminating that source of error in all cases of pyrexia suspected to be due to Yellow Fever.

(8) That the diagnostic value of albuminuria as a symptom of Yellow Fever remains unimpaired.

(*C*) The Diagnostic Significance of the Presence of Malaria Parasites and Pigmented Leucocytes in the Blood in Cases of Pyrexia, and of their Absence.

The importance of an examination of the blood for malarial parasites and pigmented leucocytes in all cases of fever in tropical countries is generally recognised, but as to the inferences to be drawn from their presence or absence, as regards the diagnosis of the disease from which the patient is suffering, there is not the same general agreement.

It will probably be useful to state first the broad facts as to the distribution of the parasites in the peripheral blood and in the organs in the various types of malarial pyrexia, in order to make the points at issue clear to those whose work has not lain specially in this branch of medicine.

The following extracts are from an article entitled "A Study of Some Fatal Cases of Malaria," by L. F. Barker, contained in the Johns Hopkins Hospital Reports:—

> "Since the discovery of Laveran's parasite, which rendered possible, under ordinary circumstances, the early recognition of a malarial infection by means of the microscopical examination of the fresh blood, it has become a comparatively rare occurrence for a patient to die of this disease. 1896, Vol V., pp. 221, 2
>
> "The study of the pathology of malaria is consequently limited to the few instances in which the patients die from traumatism, or from some intercurrent disease, and to those rare cases of pernicious malarial infection which terminate fatally."

In a separate section "On the unequal distribution of the parasites in the body in malarial infection" contained in the same paper, the following occurs:— *Ibid*, p. 26

> "* * * * * * the broad statement may be made that in infections with quartan parasites one sees the most equal distribution of the parasites throughout the blood and various organs, and that in infections with parasites of the æstivo-autumnal variety the most unequal distribution is encountered. In infection with parasites of the tertian type the character of the distribution may be said to stand between that of the quartan and that of the æstivo-autumnal infections, approaching perhaps a little more closely to the former.
>
> "In the quartan fevers the parasites are nearly always to be seen in numbers in the blood in any of the peripheral parts * * * * * *."
>
> "The parasites in tertian fever, although usually quite abundant in the circulating blood, show decidedly a more marked tendency to accumulate in the internal organs, such as the spleen, the liver and the marrow of bones. This is notably true at the time of the paroxysms, when the segmenting organisms, although usually still present in severe infections in considerable numbers in the peripheral blood, are for the most part retained in the internal organs and especially in the spleen. But it is in the infections with the æstivo-autumnal parasites, infections which include the majority of comatose and other pernicious cases, that the most curious and marked variations in the distribution of the parasites are to be met with * * * * * *.
>
> "In the æstivo-autumnal infections the number of organisms circulating in the peripheral parts affords, as a rule, very indifferent data upon which to base an idea of the severity of the infection. * * * * * * numerous slides prepared from the peripheral blood may

show very few organisms, and these often of the type most difficult to recognise, while in a drop of blood taken from the spleen quite a large number of the parasites may often be made out with ease.

"The occurrence of segmenting organisms in the peripheral blood is a phenomenon of extreme rarity in æstivo-autumnal infections."

It may, however, be noted that punctures of the spleen during life have not shewn that when the malarial parasites are scanty in the blood they *must* be numerous in internal organs.

We are now in a position to state the points at issue, viz.:—

(1) Under what circumstances does the finding of malaria parasites in the blood justify a diagnosis of Malaria?

(2) Under what circumstances does the absence of parasites from the peripheral blood negative a diagnosis of Malaria?

It is perhaps unnecessary to state that the diagnosis in any case of disease is the opinion arrived at, after a consideration of all the facts of the case, as to the nature of the malady from which the patient is suffering.

In dealing with a native population saturated with Malaria, such as that of the West African Colonies, and with malaria-infected Europeans living there, it is certain that the parasites of that disease will be found in many patients who are not suffering at the time from Malaria, although they are harbouring the organisms.

It is also important to remember the length of time after infection that the parasites may remain in the body and their capacity for lying latent during long periods.

We may illustrate the point by reference to the description contained in the Second Report of the Commission of what occurred immediately preceding the acceptance by all concerned of the diagnosis of Yellow Fever in the Ocean Springs Epidemic, Mississippi, in 1897. This epidemic started with a large number of mild and unrecognised cases, variously estimated at from 500 to 700, and during its official continuance included 4,426 cases with a mortality of 494.

"The record of the final interview between the Federal and the State officials, when the diagnosis of Yellow Fever was still being resisted and the tension extreme, is almost dramatic. Just as relations were about to be broken off and the Marine Hospital Service officers had decided to leave, 'the resident physician hastily announced the imminent death from convulsions of Miss Shutze, the patient seen by Dr. Saunders and diagnosed as Yellow Fever. This information was a thunderclap to those who had announced it Dengue.'

"It is interesting to note that the case on which the diagnosis of Yellow Fever was finally accepted by all was one in which that disease proved fatal in an individual previously infected with Malaria, and in whose blood the malarial parasites were found shortly before death. They were present in four out of five cases of the fever then again specially examined, but it is not stated that the other cases were fatal."

This occurrence sufficiently illustrates the fact that all patients in whose blood malarial organisms are found are not necessarily suffering from that disease alone. They may, as in the case just mentioned, be ill with Yellow Fever. It is a good example of the danger of relying upon laboratory tests to the exclusion of clinical experience.

We have now to consider whether there are circumstances under which a diagnosis of Malaria is justified, notwithstanding the absence of parasites from the peripheral blood.

It is obvious that if they can always, or nearly always, be found in cases of Malaria in which the symptoms are severe, their absence in any case of serious illness tells very decidedly against a diagnosis of Malaria.

Similarly, if they can always, or nearly always, be found in cases of Malaria of the type which simulates Yellow Fever, their absence tends to exclude Malaria as a possible diagnosis.

It is therefore a matter of great importance to decide when they are commonly present and when they may be absent.

These points are to some extent dealt with in the quotation from Dr. Barker's article, but further evidence is necessary.

It will be remembered that in discussing the occurrence of albuminuria in Malaria (*vide* p. 172) reference was made to the fact that in 616 cases of Malaria treated in the Johns Hopkins Hospital, between the years 1889 and 1894, Thayer and Hewetson found the parasite in every acute case of that disease admitted to the wards.

Lt.-Colonel Statham in the article to which reference has previously been made (*vide* Investigators' Reports Vol. II., p. 377) discusses this question as follows:—

"2. The great difficulty occasionally met with is in finding parasites in cases which are clinically typical malarias. This difficulty is comprehensible when the immune West African is in question, but in a West Indian or European soldier this difficulty is also often encountered, and the parasite is only found after hours, or even days, of searching, though no quinine may have been taken, and periodicity allowed for. I have had similar difficulty with subtertian malaria in South Africa, but cannot remember such cases in India.

"This difficulty of demonstrating the parasite in some cases may account for some of the cases in the group labelled 'Probable Malaria' in Table XL, though it has to be admitted that in the majority of these cases only one blood examination was carried out. It may also account for some of the cases in the 'Pyrexia with enteritis' group and in the 'Pyrexia of uncertain origin' group, where some of the clinical symptoms pointed to malaria, but no parasites could be found."

r and rae—"A em of icine;" le, alaria." I, p. 422.

McCrae, in the article from which we have already quoted under "Symptoms of Quotidian Æstivo-Autumnal Infections," states:—

"The temperature curve in the quotidian form is not characteristic, as it resembles very closely that of double tertian infection, and we must therefore depend upon the microscope in making our diagnosis. There is no greater proof of the value of a microscopic examination of the blood than is found in the ease with which the various forms of malarial fever may be diagnosed and differentiated by it."

Again:—

"In a fatal case (of the comatose form) observed by the writer, the temperature never went above 101° F., until a few hours before death, when it rose to 103° F., the entire attack lasting six days. In this case the disease was not recognised by the attending physician until a few hours before death, when a blood examination was asked for and large numbers of quotidian æstivo-autumnal parasites were found."

, p. 425.

In the same article under "The Irregular and Intermittent Forms" we read:—

"An examination of the blood, if carefully made and repeated if necessary, will invariably demonstrate the type of malarial parasite concerned, which is generally one of the æstivo-autumnal organisms."

, p. 427.

Again, under "Latent and Masked Infections":—

"A latent malarial infection may be defined as one in which parasites can be demonstrated in the blood, but in which there are no symptoms which would lead a clinician to suspect malaria, whilst a masked infection is one in which the symptoms are obscured by some accompanying disease, or in which they are atypical in character."

"At the United States Army General Hospital in San Francisco, California, out of 1,267 cases of malaria in which the parasites were demonstrated in the blood, 395 or 25 per cent. have shown either latent or masked infections.

"The æstivo-autumnal infections comprised 275 of the cases, thus showing that the æstivo-autumnal parasite is concerned most often in latent and masked malaria. Examinations of the blood in such cases have shown the parasites in all stages of development, but always in small numbers. Of the 395 cases, 277 were latent infections, or infections in which the malarial parasites could be demonstrated in the blood, but which presented no clinical symptoms, while 118 were masked infections, most of them being in patients suffering from other diseases which masked the malarial symptoms. Of the masked infections, chronic dysentery, chronic diarrhœa, pulmonary tuberculosis and amœbic dysentery were the diseases which most often masked the malarial infections."

It may be remarked, in passing, that these were the diseases from which the patients were suffering; the malarial symptoms may have been masked, or there may have been no malarial symptoms to mask.

And again:—

"*Examination of the blood.*—In most instances one examination of the blood will be sufficient, but if a negative result is obtained repeated examinations should be made at short intervals. If this is done, almost invariably, even in the most obscure æstivo-autumnal infections, the parasites will be discovered. *Ibid*, p. 43

"Cases of malaria of this variety undoubtedly occur in which no parasites can be discovered in the peripheral blood, *but not when the infection is severe enough to produce symptoms.* (The italics are not in original.)

"The symptoms in æstivo-autumnal infections are often so obscure or even so slight *that malaria is not suspected, and in many cases an examination of the blood will show the presence of the malarial plasmodia before any clinical symptoms sufficiently severe to excite a suspicion that the infection existed.* It follows then that an examination of the blood in all cases of disease occurring in malarious localities should be adopted as a routine measure." (Italics are in the origi[nal].)

The above statements lend no support to the view that a large number of cases of severe illness of sudden onset with marked pyrexia, and albuminuria, cases which may indeed end fatally in a few days, but in which no malarial organisms have been found after repeated examinations of the blood, may yet be due to Malaria.

Sir Leonard Rogers, in his work on "Fevers in the Tropics," writes as follows:— Second Edition, p. 220.

"TABLE XXIII.—NUMBER OF MALARIAL PARASITES FOUND IN 200 CASES.

	Malignant Tertians.		Benign Tertians.		Totals.		
Very numerous	20	(1)	35	(4)	56	(5)	} 78 per cent.
Numerous ...	54	(7)	46	(3)	100	(10)	
Rather few ...	9	(4)	12	(0)	21	(4)	
Very few ...	13	(9)	7	(2)	20	(11)	10 per cent.
Crescents only	3	(1)	—	-	3	(1)	

"Very numerous = Parasites found immediately.

"Numerous = Parasites found after a very short search, one minute or less.

"Rather few = Parasites found up to five minutes.

"Very few = Occasional parasites after five to ten minutes' search.

"In 78 per cent. the parasites were sufficiently numerous to allow of their detection within a minute or two.

"In only 10 per cent. were they so few as to necessitate over five minutes' search.

"The figures in the brackets indicate the number of cases in which quinine was known to have been taken before the blood was examined, while this was also doubtless the case with some others in which the point had not been noted. They show that although the parasites may be found in large numbers after some quinine has been taken, yet as a rule they are few in number after its administration; no less than 11 out of the 20 cases with 'very few' parasites had been noted to have previously taken the drug. If these are excluded, then the parasites were 'very few' in only 5 per cent. of the remainder. On the other hand, cases which are undoubtedly malarial clinically are met with in which no parasites are found at a single examination of the blood. It is difficult to accurately estimate their proportion, but a careful study of my two years' records has led me to the conclusion that they constitute between 10 and 20 per cent. of the total number of malarial fevers seen, the majority of the patients having taken quinine before admission, but most of them can readily be recognised by clinical methods, and especially by the temperature curves of four-hour charts. The absence of the parasites, then, should not be taken as evidence of the case not being malarial if it presents the typical characters of that disease, especially if quinine has been taken before the microscopical examination."

). 226. The same author states under "Complications of Malaria":—

"*Cerebral Malaria*:—

"* * * * * *. It only occurs in very intense infections, as in the case already mentioned, from which the later stages of the malignant tertian parasites of the coloured plate were drawn * * * * * *. Now during this complication of malaria (which by the way is almost always of the malignant tertian form) the parasites are so numerous in the peripheral blood that they are seen in every field of the microscope, so that they can be found easily within five minutes, including the staining of the slide."

Dr. Deeks, Chief of the Medical Clinic in the Ancon Hospital, kindly gave evidence at one of the meetings of the Commission, and was specially questioned on the diagnosis of Malaria, a disease of which he has had large experience, and Yellow Fever. In his opinion Malaria parasites were always found in severe cases of the æstivo-autumnal type, provided they had not been treated with quinine, and it was cases of that type which most often resembled Yellow Fever. He thought there was no difficulty in distinguishing between cases of that kind and Yellow Fever, if the microscope was used.

Major Perry, of the Sanitary Department, Panama Canal Zone, who attended at the same meeting, was also of opinion that there was no practical difficulty in distinguishing between cases of Malaria of the type under discussion and of Yellow Fever.

The inferences* to be drawn from the foregoing and other evidence, so far only as the question of the presence of malarial parasites is concerned, would appear to be:—

(1) That in nearly all severe untreated cases of æstivo-autumnal Malaria with pyrexia, parasites are present.

(2) That if quinine in considerable doses has been given it may be difficult to find parasites, though in practically all cases they can be found by means of Ross's thick film method (*vide* p. 167).

(3) That after heroic doses of quinine, in cases which afterwards terminate fatally, parasites may not be discovered until the post-mortem examination, and then they may only be found in certain regions, such as the brain and spleen, and even in those situations they may not be numerous.

(4) That if in an untreated case of pyrexia, accompanied by bilious vomiting and jaundice, no malarial parasites are found by the thick film method, the case is almost certainly not one of Malaria.

(5) That in any untreated case of severe pyrexia of sudden onset in which no Malaria parasites are found in the peripheral blood after several careful examinations the presumption is strongly against a diagnosis of Malaria, on that ground alone, and apart from any other consideration.

---

* Some of these inferences are stated in Doctor Deeks's own words.

(*D*) Hyperpyrexial Fever and Hyperpyrexia in Malaria and in Yellow Fever.

The investigators appointed by the Commission were instructed to pay close attention to (amongst many others) all cases of fever which might be or might resemble "(*j*) Hyperpyrexial Fever."

The following description of this disease, the nature of which is very doubtful, is taken from Sir Patrick Manson's work on "Tropical Diseases":—

> "*Symptoms.*—Thompstone and Bennett describe the clinical features thus: 'This fever is generally ushered in by a slight rise of temperature, followed by profuse perspiration and a fall in the temperature to about 99° F. After a period of apyrexia of perhaps twenty-four hours' duration, the temperature begins again to rise, slowly at first, but when 105° is passed, with alarming rapidity, one degree in ten minutes having been frequently observed, and it may reach 107° on the second day. For fourteen or even for thirty days subsequently there is absolutely no tendency for it to fall. The skin acts either very slightly or not at all, and all antipyretic drugs fail.'
>
> "In due course the tongue becomes dry and shrivelled, but the spleen and liver are not enlarged; the urine is normal and abundant, the bowels being regular or loose. The conjunctivæ are injected, the pupils contracted. There is much anxiety and restlessness; but the mind is clear in most cases except when the temperature is very high.
>
> "If the patient is to recover, a change for the better may be looked for about the end of the third week. Convalescence is very gradual, and it may be six weeks before temperature is normal. Half the cases die.
>
> "A curious feature is the remarkable rapidity with which the blood coagulates the moment it is exposed to the air.
>
> "Malaria parasites, though carefully sought for, have not been found; neither have attempts at cultivations from the blood yielded any micro-organism. The white corpuscles are rather in excess."

We are not aware that the observation of Thompstone and Bennett has been confirmed; certainly no case has been observed to which this description would apply, or in which hyperpyrexia lasted for any period approaching fourteen days, but hyperpyrexia has been a feature of a certain number of cases, most of which were diagnosed locally as either "Yellow Fever" or as "suspected Yellow Fever."

There is little doubt that on the West Coast of Africa cases have occurred in the past in which hyperpyrexia has been a very marked feature, and that such cases have been invariably reported under the heading "Malaria." Hyperpyrexia occurs in Pernicious Malaria, and some, or possibly all of them, may have been of that nature, but the measure of proof which would have been afforded by the discovery of malarial parasites in the blood and organs has very often been lacking.

Sir Patrick Manson gives the following description of the "Cerebral Form of Pernicious Malaria," in which hyperpyrexia is a marked symptom:— *Ibid*, p. 73.

> "*HYPERPYREXIAL.*—There can be little doubt that many of the cases of sudden death from hyperpyrexia and coma, usually credited to what has been called 'ardent fever' or 'heat apoplexy,' are really malarial. If careful inquiry be made into the antecedents of many of these cases, a history of mild intermittent fever will often be elicited; or it will be found that the patient had been living in some highly malarious locality.
>
> "In the course of what seemed to be an ordinary malarial attack the body temperature, instead of stopping at 104° or 105° F., may continue to rise and, passing 107°, rapidly mount to 110° or even to 112°. The patient, after a brief stage of wild, maniacal or, perhaps, muttering delirium, becomes rapidly unconscious, then comatose, and dies within a few hours, or perhaps within an hour, of the onset of the pernicious symptoms."

The following is the Medical Report on a case, which occurred in West Africa, of the kind described by Sir Patrick Manson:

> "CASE REPORT.
>
> "Sergt.-Major ———
>
> "*Disease:* Malaria.
>
> "*Admitted:* 8-10-13.
>
> "*Result:* Death, 13-10-13.
>
> "*Cause:* Hyperpyrexia.
>
> "On the morning of Wednesday, October 8th, 1913, I was called to attend Sergt.-Major ——— in his quarters, and found him suffering from Malaria; the case was neither severe nor in any way out of the ordinary. His temperature varied from 99° to 101·4°, gradually subsiding under ordinary treatment till on Sunday it was normal. He was kept in bed, however, and when seen by me on Monday morning it was found that he had a temperature of 99·2°. He had no pain, headache, or other symptoms. His condition remained the same throughout the day, and in no way gave rise to any alarm.
>
> "Between 6.30 and 7 p.m. his temperature suddenly rose to 106° F. Cold sponging, stimulants and intramuscular injections of

quinine were resorted to, for he became slightly delirious and his pulse was weak and rapid. About 8 o'clock he became quieter, his skin became moist, and he settled down to sleep; half an hour later he died without even waking up.

"In the opinion of some of his friends, Sergt.-Major ——— had had a good deal of Malaria lately without reporting sick. I think that this is probably true, as he certainly seemed more debilitated and weaker than one would expect him to be in such a comparatively mild attack as this last one."

In the Second Report of the Commission (p. 61), in the account of the incidence of Yellow Fever in the Gambia, the following occurs:—

"1906.

"One case of remittent fever ending in malarial cachexia, and one of malignant remittent fever with hyperpyrexia. In the latter case quinine was not for some reason assimilated, though given by the mouth in large doses, the liver being at the same time acting freely, the hyperpyrexia could only be subdued by ice-packs, and intramuscular injections of quinine produced an immediate beneficial effect on the course of the fever, causing an uninterrupted convalescence to set in."

"In the case of a similar nature previously reported in detail (1899) it was clear that the ice-packs and not the quinine caused the fall of temperature. The exact nature of these cases is doubtful."

Vol. I., , seq.

The "Report on certain outbreaks of Yellow Fever in Lagos, 1913, and January and February, 1914," by Dr. T. M. Russell Leonard, contains an account of certain cases diagnosed as Yellow Fever, all of which occurred on board ships, and in all of which hyperpyrexia was a prominent symptom.

As some readers of this report may not possess the volume of the Investigators' Reports in which those cases are detailed, a selection of typical examples is reproduced here:—

"CASE NO. 29. L. 102.

"*Sex*: Male
"*Age*: 21 years.
"*Nationality*: European, German.
"*Occupation*: Steward.
"*Date of death*: 26th October.
"*Diagnosis after post-mortem examination*: Yellow fever.

"This case died on board the ss. '*Elizabeth Brock*,' at 7.10 a.m. on the 26th October. The body was brought ashore for an autopsy.

"*Previous history.*—This was obtained from the Captain of the vessel. The man complained of being ill on the morning of the 23rd October with headache and fever, temperature at noon that day being 103·2°, and at 8 p.m. 103·4°. Next day, the 24th, the temperature was 100·2° at 8 a.m., and 104° at 8 p.m. On the 25th the temperature fell to 99·2° and then began steadily to rise, being 103·8° at 8 p.m. that night, and next morning, the 26th, at 7 a.m., it was 106°, and the patient died at 7.10.

"Autopsy performed at the Lagos Hospital at 9 a.m.

"*Skin.*—Sallow appearance. Deep cyanosis of the ears and genital organs. No rash present.

"*Rigor mortis.*—Present.

"*Brain.*—Normal.

"*Spinal cord.*—Normal.

"*Membranes.*—Normal.

"*Heart.*—Weight, 11½ ozs. Pale and flabby. Valves normal.

"*Large vessels.*—Normal.

"*Lung, right.*—Weight, 18½ ozs. Very congested, particularly at base.

"*Lung, left.*—Weight, 17½ ozs. Congested.

"*Pleuræ.*—Normal. No adhesions. Contents, 2 ozs. yellow fluid.

"*Larynx, trachea, bronchi.*—Mucous membrane congested.

"*Peritoneum.*—Normal.

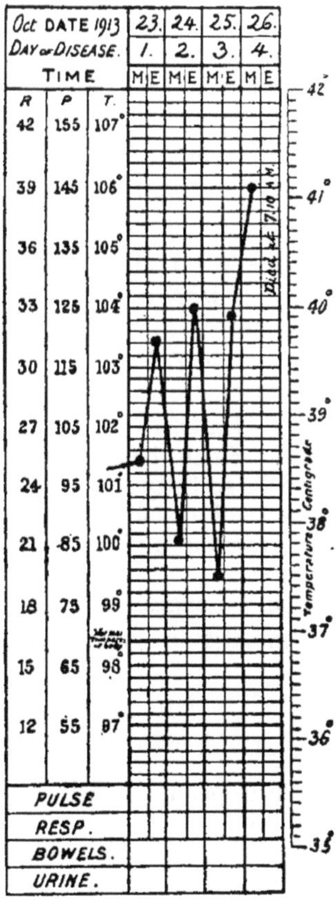

Oct DATE 1913	23.	24.	25.	26.
DAY of DISEASE.	1.	2.	3.	4.
TIME	M E	M E	M E	M E

R	P	T.	Temperature Centigrade
			42°
42	155	107°	
39	145	106°	41°
36	135	105°	
33	125	104°	40°
30	115	103°	
27	105	102°	39°
24	95	101°	
21	85	100°	38°
18	75	99°	37°
15	65	98°	
12	55	97°	36°
			35°

Died at 7.10 A.M.

PULSE
RESP.
BOWELS.
URINE.

CHART 28.

"*Stomach.*—Mucous membrane congested. Rugæ swollen. Extensive submucous hæmorrhages at the cardiac end, pylorus and posterior wall. Vessels engorged. Stomach empty, brown mucus adhering to walls.

"*Small intestine.*—Duodenum congested. Hæmorrhages present in its entire length. Jejunum also congested and hæmorrhages present. Contents, brown fluid.

"*Large intestine.*—Normal.

"*Helminths.*—None present.

"*Liver.*—Weight, 68 ozs. Congested. Hæmorrhages present under capsule. Friable. Greasy on section.

"*Gall bladder.*—Normal. Contents, 2 ozs. normal bile.

"*Pancreas.*—Normal. Weight, 6 ozs.

"*Spleen.*—Weight, 13½ ozs. Enlarged, soft and pulpy.

"*Kidney, right.*—Weight, 6½ ozs. Congested. Capsule strips easily. Stellate veins enlarged.

"*Kidney, left.*—Weight, 6½ ozs. Same appearance as right.

"*Suprarenal capsules.*—Normal.

"*Lymphatic system.*—Normal.

"*Bladder.*—Mucous membrane congested. Hæmorrhages present. Contained one teaspoonful of muddy urine. Acid in reaction Highly albuminous. Tube casts also present.

"*Diagnosis.*—Yellow fever.

"Smears from organs and specimens sent to Research Institute.

"LABORATORY REPORT.

Microscopic.

"1. Smear preparations from :—

(*a*) *Spleen.*—*Paraplasma flavigenum* present.
(*b*) *Liver.*—*Paraplasma flavigenum* present.
(*c*) *Bone marrow.*—*Paraplasma flavigenum* present.
(*d*) *Lung.*—*Paraplasma flavigenum* present.

"2. Histological :—

(*a*) *Liver.*—Extensive fatty metamorphosis. Lobules distorted. Small hæmorrhages present. Few cells contained large fatty globules.
(*b*) *Kidney.*—Fatty metamorphosis present. Tubules filled with granular and hyaline débris. Denuded of cells in places.
(*c*) *Spleen.*—Congested.

"3. Urine examination: Acid reaction. Highly albuminous. Tube casts present.

"CASE NO. 32. L. 105.

"*Sex* : Male.

"*Age* : 27 years.

"*Nationality* : European, British.

"*Occupation* : Ship's officer.

"*Date of admission* : 26th November, 1913.

"*Date of death* : 26th November, 1913.

"*Diagnosis* : Yellow fever.

"*History.*—Patient was sent into hospital at 4.15 p.m. on the 26th November from the s.s. '*Bassa.*' The patient was delirious, temperature 106·8°. The vessel had arrived from Foreados on the 24th; the man had been 'seedy' for a couple of days.

"*On admission.*—Patient wildly delirious. Face and neck cyanosed. Pulse very quick and thready. Pupils widely dilated. Passed 4 ozs. of urine after admission. Temperature in axilla, 106·8°.

"*Alimentary system.*—Liver and spleen were normal. Tongue was pointed and red.

"*Respiratory system.*—Respirations were rapid. Breathing stertorous.

"*Nervous system.*—Pupils widely dilated. Delirium present.

"*Urinary system.* Urine was clear, reddish yellow in colour. Acid reaction. Sp. gr. 1025. No albumen present. Phosphates present.

"*Skin.*—Skin was covered with a red rash. Face, neck and chest showed patches of cyanosis. Conjunctivæ very injected. Eyes shining.

"*Blood examination.*—Few malaria parasites present. *Paraplasma flavigenum* present. Differential count: Polymorphonuclear, 66·5 per cent.; mononuclear, 11·6 per cent.; lymphocytes, 18 per cent.; eosinophil, 0·5 per cent.; transitionals, 3·4 per cent. Patient was given an intramuscular injection of quinine, grs. 10. Wet pack.

"At 5.20 p.m. temperature in axilla was 106·2°. Breathing stertorous. Face and chest cyanosed. At 5.30 patient placed in ice pack, rectal temperature 108·6°. At 6 p.m. vomiting occurred, bilious in character, and took place several times. At 6.45 p.m. rectal temperature was 105·6°, pulse had improved and was 115 per minute. Breathing easier and not stertorous. Delirium stopped and patient quiet.

"At 7.45 p.m., patient in the same condition, rectal temperature 105·7°, pulse 129 per minute. Vomiting again occurred, bilious. At 8.45 p.m. patient became very restless. Rectal temperature 105·8°. Convulsions set in, and patient died at 9 p.m.

"*Post-mortem notes.*—Autopsy was performed at 8 a.m. next morning. Skin was yellow. Ears, neck and face cyanosed. Genital organs were deeply cyanosed. Conjunctivæ showed hæmorrhages.

"*Rigor mortis.*—Present.

"*Brain.*—Vessels engorged. Brain substance congested.

"*Spinal cord.*—Congested.

"*Membranes.*—Congested. Vessels engorged. Dura mater adherent to calvarium. Pia and arachnoid mater adherent to brain.

"*Heart.*—Weight 10½ ozs., pale and flabby, valves normal. Hæmorrhages present on the epicardium as well as on the endocardium of the right auricle and ventricle.

"*Large vessels.*—Normal.

"*Lung, right.*—Weight 14½ ozs., normal, some congestion at base.

"*Lung, left.*—Weight 12½ ozs., normal.

"*Pleuræ.*—Normal, no adhesions.

"*Larynx, trachea, bronchi.*—Mucous membrane, slight congestion.

"*Peritoneum.*—Normal.

"*Stomach.*—Peritoneal surface congested. Vessels engorged. Mucous membrane congested. Rugæ prominent. Large areas of hæmorrhage in the posterior wall, cardiac and pyloric ends, and along the greater curvature. Contents: 1 oz. of brown fluid.

"*Small intestine.*—Duodenum congested. Hæmorrhages present in its entire length. Jejunum and ileum presented the same condition. Contents: brown fluid.

"*Large intestine.*—Normal.

"*Helminths.*—None present.

"*Liver.*—Weight, 43 ozs., congested, with yellow patches. Friable, greasy on section. Hæmorrhages seen under capsule.

"*Gall bladder.*—Distended with normal bile.

"*Pancreas.*—Normal. Weight, $3\frac{3}{4}$ ozs.

"*Spleen.*—Weight, $6\frac{1}{2}$ ozs. Congested. Soft and pulpy.

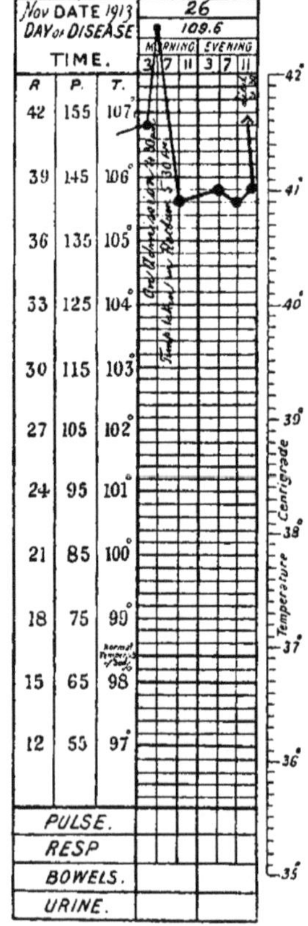

CHART 31.

"*Kidney, right.*—Weight, $5\frac{1}{2}$ ozs. Very congested. Capsule strips easily. Stellate veins prominent.

"*Kidney, left.*—Weight, $5\frac{1}{2}$ ozs. Same appearance as the right.

"*Suprarenal capsules.*—Normal.

"*Lymphatic system.*—Normal.

"*Bladder.*—Contracted. Mucous membrane congested and showed small hæmorrhages. Contents: 3 ozs. turbid urine. Acid reaction and highly albuminous.

"LABORATORY REPORT.

"*Microscopical.*

"1. Blood smears and smears from organs.

"(*a*) *Blood.*—*Paraplasma flavigenum* present.

"(*b*) *Heart.*—*Paraplasma flavigenum* present.

"(*c*) *Spleen.*—Negative.

"(*d*) *Lung.*—*Paraplasma flavigenum* present.

"2. Histological.

"(*a*) *Liver.*—Fatty degeneration. Small hæmorrhages present.

"(*b*) *Kidney.*—Fatty degeneration present. Tubules denuded of epithelium in places. Tubules blocked with granular and hyaline débris.

"3. *Urine examination*: Acid reaction. Highly albuminous. Tube casts present."

"CASE NO. 34. L. 107.

"*Sex*: Male.

"*Age*: 41 years.

"*Nationality*: European, British.

"*Occupation*: Steward.

"*Date of death*: 24th December, 1913.

"*Diagnosis after post-mortem*: Yellow fever.

"*History.*—The following history of the case was obtained from the Captain of the vessel, as the patient had died on the way to the hospital. The deceased had been 'seedy' for the previous two days, but had not complained. On the morning of the 24th he complained that he felt feverish, and, his temperature being taken, it was found to be 104°. He went to bed and a doctor was sent for. He was quite sensible and had taken some beef tea. Dr. Gray saw him at 3 p.m., and found him quite unconscious, with stertorous breathing, and with an axillary temperature of 109°. He advised his immediate removal to hospital, and death took place on the way.

"POST-MORTEM NOTES.

"The autopsy was performed at 5 p.m. that evening. Face, ears and neck were cyanosed. Patches of petechial eruption present on the abdomen and thighs. Genital organs cyanosed. Body was well nourished and fat.

"*Rigor mortis.*—Had not begun.

"*Brain.*—Vessels engorged. Brain substance congested.

"*Spinal cord.*—Congested.

"*Membranes.*—Vessels engorged. Membranes adherent.

"*Heart.*—Weight, 13 ozs. Pale and flabby. Valves normal.

"*Large vessels.*—Aorta showed a patch of atheroma.

"*Lung, right.*—Weight, 16 ozs. Congested at base.

"*Lung, left.*—Weight, 17 ozs. Very congested at base.

"*Pleuræ.*—Normal. No adhesions.

"*Larynx, trachea, bronchi.*—Mucous membrane congested.

"*Peritoneum.*—Normal. Very fatty.

"*Stomach.*—Peritoneal surface congested. Vessels prominent and engorged. Mucous membrane congested. Rugæ swollen. Hæmorrhages present at cardiac and pyloric ends, also on posterior wall and along the greater curvature. Stomach was empty.

"*Small intestine.*—Duodenum congested. Hæmorrhages present in its entire length. Jejunum also congested and submucous hæmorrhages present. Ileum congested.

"*Large intestine.*—Normal.

"*Helminths.*—None present.

"*Liver.*—Weight, 82 ozs. Left lobe yellow. Right lobe very congested. Hæmorrhages present under capsule. Very friable. Greasy on section.

"*Gall bladder.*—Normal.

"*Pancreas.*—Weight, 5 ozs. Normal.

"*Spleen.*—Weight, 4 ozs. Soft and pulpy.

"*Kidney, right.*—Weight, 7 ozs. Congested. Capsule strips readily. Cortex congested.

"*Kidney, left.*—Weight, 7½ ozs. Very congested. Capsule strips easily.

"*Suprarenal capsule.*—Normal.

"*Lymphatic system.*—Normal.

"*Bladder.*—Normal. Contained 3 ozs. of urine. Urine was acid in reaction and albuminous.

"LABORATORY REPORT.

"*Microscopical.*

"1. Blood and smears from organs:—

"(*a*) *Blood*: *Paraplasma flavigenum* present.

"(*b*) *Spleen*: Negative.

"(*c*) *Liver*: *Paraplasma flavigenum* present.

"(*d*) *Kidney*: Negative.

"2. Histological:—

"(*a*) *Liver*: Fatty degeneration present and extensive. Hæmorrhages present.

"(*b*) *Spleen*: Normal.

"(*c*) *Kidney*: Fatty metamorphosis. Tubules filled with granular and hyaline débris. Cells of convoluted tubules swollen and granular.

"3. Urine examination: Acid reaction. Albumen present. Tube casts also present."

"CASE NO. 35. L. 119.

"*Notes by Dr. Manson.*

"*Sex*: Male.

"*Age*: ——.

"*Nationality*: European, British.

"*Occupation*: Ship's officer.

"*Date of death*: 28th December, 1913.

"*Diagnosis after post-mortem*: Yellow fever.

"Dr. Manson reports that he was called to see this patient on the afternoon of the 28th, the vessel lying in the Lagos Roads. On his arrival he found the patient unconscious and in convulsions, and death occurred in his presence about 5 p.m.

"The following history was obtained from the captain of the vessel. The deceased had complained of fever on the 25th December, and his temperature was 102°. On the 26th, at 10 a.m., it was 103°. On the 27th the morning temperature was 103°, and at 6 p.m. it had risen to 105·4°. On the 28th at 2 a.m. it was 105·4°, at 9 a.m. 103·4°, and at 4 p.m. it had risen to 106°. At 4.30 p.m. patient had vomited some black-looking fluid. Temperature taken just before death was 106°, and the pulse rate 70.

"POST-MORTEM NOTES.

"Autopsy was performed by Dr. Manson at 7 a.m. next morning.

"*Rigor mortis* was well marked. Petechial patches on the neck and chest. Genital organs cyanosed.

"*Kidneys.*—Enlarged. Capsules strip easily.

"*Spleen.*—Enlarged and soft.

"*Liver.*—Size normal, paler than normal.

"*Stomach and duodenum.*—Removed *en masse.* Stomach contained some greenish-black fluid which looked like altered blood. Hæmorrhages present in the M. membrane of the greater part of the stomach and duodenum.

"*Bladder.*—Contracted but contained a small amount of urine, which was drawn off and on testing was found to contain albumen.

"Portions of spleen, liver and kidney, together with smears and the whole of the stomach and duodenum, were sent to the Medical Research Institute, Yaba, for further examination and report.

"*Diagnosis.*—Yellow fever.

"*Laboratory Report.*—None received.

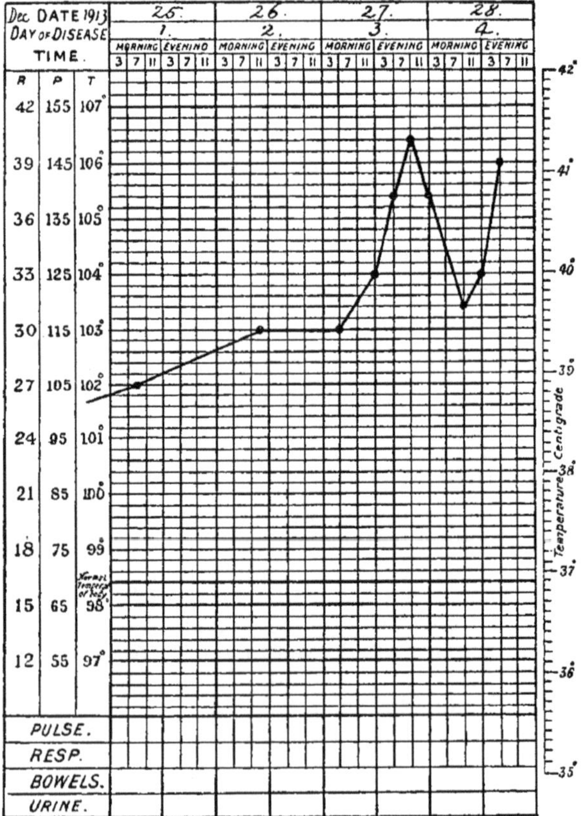

CHART 32.

"NOTE.—With the exception of the pulse record on the day of death (made by the Medical Officer, Lagos), this chart was compiled from observations made by the captain of the vessel.

"According to the captain's statement the pulse-rate had never been more than 80 per minute."

In each of these cases, although the evidence is defective in certain important particulars, it is, we think, difficult to arrive at any other diagnosis than that of Yellow Fever, which was the opinion formed by the medical officers, who either saw the case or made the post-mortem or pathological examination. If this view is correct, the cases are sufficient to establish the fact that hyperpyrexia may be a feature of Yellow Fever, and that a careful examination of the blood is necessary in all such cases before it is concluded that they are cases of Malaria. The defects in the evidence are due to the fact that all the cases occurred on board ship.

The following case is of great interest, and there is no doubt room for difference of opinion as to its nature:—

"CASE NO. 37.

"*Sex*: Male.

"*Age*: No record.

"*Nationality*: European, British.

"*Occupation*: Ship's officer.

"*Date of death*: 23rd October, 1913.

"The following report of this case was sent in by the surgeon of the vessel:—

"'On Monday, the 20th of October, at 10.40 a.m., the deceased reported sick. On examination, I found that his temperature was 105°, no headache or any other symptom complained of. He was placed in hospital on the ship, phenacetin and caffeine being administered. Diet: Milk and soda. Temperature became normal about 11 p.m., when 20 grains of quinine were given by the rectum, patient being unable to take quinine by mouth.

"'From above date and hour (11 p.m.) temperature remained normal until the evening of the 22nd, when it rose to 101°, but was reduced at 11 p.m. to normal.

"'On the morning of the 23rd I was sent for by the night attendant at the hospital. I found the patient slightly delirious, head very hot, temperature 103°. I placed calves of legs in flannel steeped in mustard and water and administered brandy, heart's action being very weak. Temperature rising at 6 a.m. to

104° and delirium increasing, I blistered behind the ears. At 7.15 a.m. temperature was 106·5°. I had a consultation with

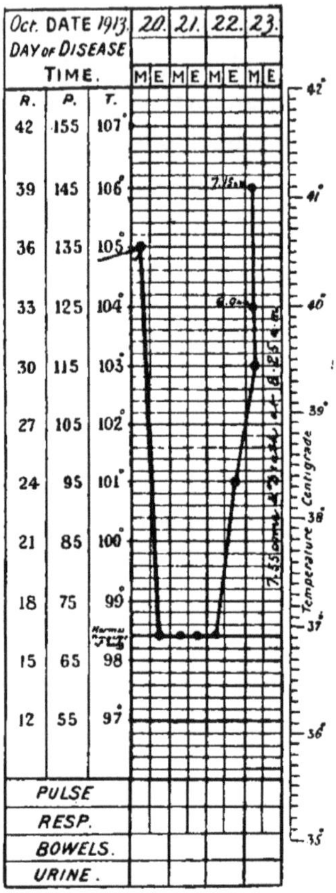

CHART 34.

Dr. O'Keeffe, Medical Officer, Government Service. Mustard was placed beneath heart and strychnine injected, but without avail, patient became comatose at 7.55 and passed away at 8.25 a.m.

"'*Diagnosis.*—Hyperpyrexia during malarial fever.'

"This case is one that must be viewed with great suspicion, as being one of yellow fever and not simple malarial fever. Unfortunately, there are no data on which any reliance can be placed in order to permit of a diagnosis being made from the above report. There are no records of blood examination, urine examination, pulse rate, and finally no post-mortem examination was made of the body in order to confirm the diagnosis. The deceased became ill in Foreados, a port in which yellow fever was known to exist. Illness was very sudden, temperature high, and vomiting apparently was present, as quinine could not be taken by the mouth. Presuming that the quinine treatment was carried on during the two days preceding death, there seems to be no reason for the hyperpyrexia, delirium, coma and death other than that the illness was complicated with yellow fever as well as malaria, as, from my experience of malarial fevers in West Africa and in the West Indies, quinine properly administered cuts short the attack of malarial fever.

"Cases quoted in this report show that yellow fever can exist side by side in the same individual as malarial fever, and in the above case there seems to be very little doubt that the cause of death was yellow fever."

The following sentence in the surgeon's report is deplorably vague:—

"Temperature became normal about 11 p.m., when 20 grains of quinine were given by the rectum, patient being unable to take quinine by mouth."

This probably means, as Dr. Leonard suggests, that the patient had been vomiting previously to 11 p.m.

Whether by "when," the writer meant to convey that 20 grains of quinine were given "about 11 p.m.," or that "when 20 grains of quinine were given by the rectum the temperature became normal," is very doubtful. The fact that the temperature fell to normal on the 20th October at 11 p.m. and remained normal until the evening of October 22nd, "when it rose to 101°, but was reduced (it is not stated by what means) at 11 p.m. to normal," is clear evidence that the case was not one of uncomplicated Yellow Fever; indeed, it is strong presumptive evidence against it being Yellow Fever at all. It will be observed that there is no statement that when the surgeon was called to the case on the morning of October 23rd he administered quinine or that quinine was given at all during the period of the continued rise in the temperature which ended in the death of the patient.

If, as is suggested, the final hyperpyrexia was an expression of the presence of a Yellow Fever factor, we should not have expected that the temperature would have been so completely controlled by the quinine, as it certainly was. It appears more probable that the quinine was not given up to the end.

(*E*) Uto-Enyin, Bayloo and Bonke.

The Commission have received a considerable amount of evidence pointing to the existence in some of the West African Dependencies of a febrile disease known to the natives by the names Uto-Enyin,

Bayloo and Bonke. The word Uto-Enyin means "yellow eyes," and jaundice appears to be one of the most common symptoms of the disease. It may be that Uto-Enyin is really Yellow Fever, of the comparatively mild type, which is its most common manifestation amongst the natives, but further investigation of this disease is necessary. It is quite possible that one or other of these names is used by the natives to describe a variety of diseases attended by fever and jaundice, one of which is no doubt Malaria.

"In September, 1910, Mr. C. Punch, District Commissioner, and Dr. A. H. Wilson, Medical Officer, were deputed to investigate the allegation that ill effects from excessive drinking were apparent in certain districts between the Calabar and Cross River. The evidence collected, while showing that excessive drinking did not obtain amongst the peoples visited, discovered that the population of the various towns and villages had decreased to a very considerable extent. The cause of this, in the opinion of nearly all the chiefs who were consulted, was a disease called Uto-Enyin. Nearly 200 people in 18 towns and villages had died from this disease during the ten months preceding the investigation. In one compound there had been 30 deaths in ten months out of a total of 400 persons; in another 20 deaths out of 700, and in yet another 18 deaths in one month out of 700 people.

"The description, as given by the different chiefs, closely corresponds, and the following is an account. It may occur in two forms, 'male and female,' the 'male' type being acute and lasting a week or ten days and ending in death or recovery; the 'female' type being more subacute or chronic and lasting one to two months, leaving the patient weak and debilitated; all ages are affected, and both sexes. One attack affords no protection against another. The same person may have as many as three or four or even six separate attacks. The onset appears to be more or less sudden, with weakness (fever). Pains are specially noted in the joints, the sides of the chest, the back of the neck and small of the back. After about two or three days jaundice appears; the eyes and finger nails become yellow, also the urine, which in very severe cases may become very dark. Vomiting and cough may be present occasionally, but are not characteristic; there is neither rash, diarrhœa nor abdominal symptoms. A severe case may end in death in five or six days. The sickness is not contagious, and the natives do not fear it in this respect."

"In 1910 Dr. Collet, S.M.O., of Sierra Leone, formerly of Southern Nigeria, on reading Dr. Wilson's report, recognised the group of symptoms and sequelæ described therein as a disease called by various names by the natives of Southern Nigeria. The Efik people of the Calabar District called the disease Uto-Enyin; other names are Akum, Obogu, Ebah, Ahuoku, Ibun and Atridi. He does not, however, consider that there are sufficient grounds for looking on the disease as a modified occurrence of yellow fever, or even a disease *sui generis*. He found that the disease was known amongst the Ibo, Ijaw, Bonny, Brass and New Calabar peoples as well as the Yorubas

He agrees that the morbid condition is an entity, but says that the supervention of jaundice in the course of an acute febrile disease is a matter of fairly frequent occurrence. In his opinion a certain proportion of the cases are simple malarial infections of the gastric type, in which there is more or less pronounced nausea with jaundice. Others prove to be gastric catarrh, obstructive jaundice, liver disorders, and in one case in his experience, pneumonia.

"He also considered that the promiscuous use of native bush medicines, if not actually responsible for the jaundice, at any rate in some cases assisted in its production, while the heroic doses of tartrate of antimony and santonin taken by many natives might occasionally induce jaundice.

"He does not preclude the possibility of the existence of a separate disease, or its connection with yellow fever in 'bayloo,' and thinks that the possible occurrence of epidemic jaundice should not be lost sight of."

"In December, 1910, Dr. T. M. Russell Leonard reported four cases of the disease, which is known among the natives of Calabar as 'yellow eyes' or 'yellow fever.' The cases were all admitted into and treated in the native hospital at Calabar. The prominent symptom in all of them was jaundice; there was severe malaise, enlargement of the spleen and liver, associated with tenderness. Vomiting of a bilious character was also present, and the bowels were constipated, except in one case, where diarrhœa was present. The blood examination showed that all these cases were purely *malaria of the bilious remittent type, the blood showing malignant tertian parasites in various stages of growth.* The urine was dark coloured, due to bile present in it. *No albumen was found in any case*, showing that the kidneys were unaffected, nor was there any hæmoglobin or blood débris present. This in itself was sufficient, in Dr. Leonard's opinion, to show that these cases were purely malarial in origin and not true 'yellow fever,' in which the presence of albumen in the urine was an important and diagnostic sign. Dr. Leonard has had experience of yellow fever in the West Indies."

"In 1911 a report was received from Dr. R. H. Kennan, Senior Sanitary Officer, Sierra Leone, containing an account of his observations on a certain disease called 'bayloo' by the Mendis, which, as described by them, bears a resemblance to yellow fever. He suggested that it may be proved to be yellow fever in an endemic form.

"This disease, according to Dr. Kennan, 'affects both adults and children, but chiefly the latter. It is believed to be infectious through contagion conveyed by the urine to persons passing over places where it has been passed on the ground or deposited. Cases arise 'one one' (*i.e.*, singly, not in epidemics like small-pox). Its prevalence is most marked at the end of the dry season (and (?) at the very early rains). The onset is sudden with acute febrile symptoms and vomiting of yellow material which may later be green, and the urine is described as 'red,' 'dark' or 'brown.' Prostration to a variable degree supervenes. In from four to seven days, or later, the 'eyes' *and finger tips under the nails become yellow*, and the diagnosis is established; but it is not pretended that the diagnosis can be made till this yellowness appears, *i.e.*, the bilious vomit and 'dark' urine are not by themselves pathognomonic. Food is not desired in the early stages, and what may be taken is usually rejected. The disease has sometimes a fatal termination, but if treatment is resorted to early, recovery is the rule. The duration of the illness varies from about ten days in children to perhaps a month or more in adults. Opinion varies in different places as to whether the same person can have the disease more than once. In some places at least it is recognised that yellowness alone (*i.e.*, without the acute symptoms having preceded it) does not justify the diagnosis of 'bayloo.' At no place was it described as the most prevalent disease or the one which caused the greatest mortality. It was in each place believed to have been 'always' in the country, and I could not find that any tradition exists regarding its first appearance. One narrator described it as a 'god's sickness,' which expression would fairly accurately describe the British matron's idea of measles, chicken-pox, or whooping cough in England.

"Inquiries were made at Mano, Bañma, Segbwema, Kasama, Pendembu, Upper Sama, Sumbuya, Tikonko, and at all these places the people knew the disease, and though the descriptions of the native chiefs vary a little in minor details, they all agree as to the main characteristics.

"Dr. Kennan understood from information obtained from some Timnehs that they knew 'bayloo' in their country by the name of 'bonkie.' He thinks that other names, such as 'wayloo,' 'burra,' etc., describe the same disease."

"In 1913 Dr. McConaghy, of Sierra Leone, reported on four cases of 'bayloo' (known amongst the Timnehs as 'bonke'). The chief symptoms were fever, vomiting, jaundice, pains in the back and legs, and 'red' eyes (by which the patients mean yellow).

"*Malaria parasites were not found.* The vomit is described as red, so are the eyes and the urine. In the cases examined *albumen was not found* at the time of examination.

"The signs and symptoms differed somewhat in the cases seen. The following were noticed:—Pains in the limbs and back, vomiting, *jaundice of the conjunctivæ and nails*, furred tongue, sometimes clean at the tip and edges, enlarged spleen in one case and enlarged liver in two; in one case jaundice was not present. There did not seem to have been any epigastric or abdominal tenderness in any of the cases. In Cases 2 and 3 the urine was actually red. In one case vomiting did not occur until the sixth day, and jaundice did not appear until the tenth, after the pains in the back and limbs had commenced."*

It is, we think, quite clear that in the cases described by Dr. Leonard the disease was Malaria; the presence of malarial parasites in various stages of growth in the blood, and, still more

* The above abstract of the evidence contained in various despatches was prepared by Dr. H. L. Burgess, Medical Secretary of the Commission.

important, the absence of albumen in the urine, negative a diagnosis of Yellow Fever.

It will, however, be noticed that in the cases reported by Dr. McConaghy, malarial parasites were not found in the blood, but again the urine, in the cases in which it was examined, was free from albumen. As we know that in mild cases of Yellow Fever albuminuria is as constant a symptom as in those of a severe type, these cases can therefore also be excluded.

There is, however, one definite point of contact between Yellow Fever and this disease or these diseases, viz., the yellow staining of the finger nails.

It will be remembered (*vide* Sporadic Cases, Section VII., p. 72) that in the case of Dr. Lundie, West African Medical Staff, who suffered from Yellow Fever at Bole, in 1913, this condition was present, and persisted during convalescence and up to the time of his arrival in London. The nails of the right hand showed hæmorrhages into the matrices, and faint traces of the same were observed in one or two nails of the left. As the nails grew the yellow stains were carried to the tips. Roughly speaking, the stains took about two months to disappear, leaving the nails thinner and with a tendency to split at the end. There was no transverse depression, as is so often observed in Pneumonia and other severe illnesses.

Dr. Mugliston, who went to Dr. Lundie's assistance at Bole, also developed Yellow Fever, but fortunately recovered. In his case the nails were not affected.

Dr. Kennan and Dr. McConaghy also mention the yellow staining of the finger nails in the cases seen by them.

Conclusions.

The following conclusions appear to be justified as to some of the epidemiological and clinical features of this disease (or ? of these diseases):—

1. That it occurs in a sporadic form and also in epidemics.
2. That at least two different types of attack are recognisable.
3. That one may cause death in five or six days.
4. That the other may assume a sub-acute or chronic form.

5. That the onset is sudden with acute febrile symptoms.

6. That all ages and both sexes are affected.

7. That it may be attended with a high mortality.

8. That in some places it is recognized that one attack affords no protection against another, whereas in other places opinion is divided upon the question.

9. That the finger nails may become yellow.

10. That the most constant symptoms are:—

(*a*) Pyrexia.

(*b*) Malaise.

(*c*) Prostration.

(*d*) Pains in various parts of the body.

(*e*) Jaundice.

(*f*) A dark colour of the urine.

(*g*) Vomiting.

11. That some, at least, of the cases are due to malarial infection.

(*F*) Weil's Disease.

This disease, which was described by Weil as occurring in Germany, may closely resemble a mild attack of Yellow Fever. Jaundice is of constant occurrence, appearing about the same period of the illness as Yellow Fever—namely, the fourth, fifth, or sixth day, and the post-mortem signs are in many respects alike. It seems to be a Septicæmia, in which the jaundice is due to a degeneration of the liver cells, and the nephritis to the injury caused to the cells of the kidney. In Weil's disease, however, a bacillus of the proteus group was found in the spleen, liver, and kidneys of two fatal cases, and in the urine of several cases during life.

SECTION XII.

MORBID ANATOMY.

No attempt will be made in this section to give a complete description of the morbid anatomy of Yellow Fever; such a labour is unnecessary, as the subject is fully dealt with in the text books and in the articles on Yellow Fever in the various systems of medicine.

The organs chiefly affected are the liver, the stomach and intestines and the kidneys; of these interest centres around the changes in the liver, owing to the recent claim of Da Rocha Lima to have demonstrated lesions therein which are characteristic of the disease.

There is not, as a rule, in cases of Yellow Fever submitted to post-mortem examination, much difficulty in deciding that the patient has died of that disease, but as the decision in sporadic cases, and in the early days of a threatened epidemic, may be a matter of such supreme importance, the discovery of a pathognomonic lesion of the liver would necessarily be a step in advance.

THE LIVER.

Macroscopic Appearances.

The following description of the appearances presented by the liver in Yellow Fever is taken from the late Sir Robert Boyce's work on "Yellow Fever and its Prevention":—

> "The *liver* is invariably altered in colour: most frequently it presents some shade of yellow, usually *boxwood* colour, but shades like bath-brick, tan, ochreous brown, deep yellow, pale yellow and reddish yellow are frequently recorded. The fact that there is *some shade of yellow*, with, in addition, some degree of *congestion*, the latter may be so pronounced that the liver looks like a yellow 'nutmeg liver.' Most observers agree that the term boxwood covers most accurately the shade of yellow which is most frequently seen. It is not a bright yellow such as is sometimes seen in jaundice. The neck of the gall bladder may be congested: this was seen in the autopsies made in Seccondee this year, 1910."

Sir Robert Boyce, 'Yellow Fever and i Prevention, p. 228.

Carrol describes the liver as:—

> "Tense, firm and smooth, showing that its cells are swollen. The colour of the organ is variable. It may be uniform or mottled in appearance, but it is always yellowish or brownish in colour, and usually shows areas of congestion or hæmorrhages beneath the capsule. Upon section the organ is firm, pale and friable. The cut surface may also be uniform or mottled."

Osler and McCrae, "A System Medicine," Art. "Yello Fever," p. 749.

The variations which are observed in the appearances presented by the liver are probably mainly due to conditions antecedent to the onset of the disease to the period during its course at which death occurs, and to the mode of death.

Precedent cirrhotic changes will necessarily have a marked effect, and it is a recognised fact that Yellow Fever is specially fatal in those who have drunk to excess. If all the organs show congestion the liver will share in that change; if hæmorrhage has been severe or if fatty degeneration is extreme it will be paler in colour. Probably the earlier the period at which death occurs, the less marked are the fatty changes. In some cases the liver is larger than normal, but rarely markedly so; in others it is smaller.

Microscopic Appearances.

The following is Da Rocha Lima's description of the histological changes in liver in Yellow Fever, which he regards as almost characteristic of that disease:—

rchiv. für iffe und pen giene," 16, 1912, 192-199.

> " In yellow fever I have found without exception in contrast to nearly all diseases a *marked attack on the intermediate zone*, which in most cases, even with low magnification, is recognisable as broad rings between the more or less altered peripheral and central zones. In the cases where the zonal divisions cannot be so easily distinguished, the diagnosis will yet become possible through a knowledge of the details about to be described.
>
> " To these details, to the manner in which the different histological elements are altered and arranged, I attach as great a value as upon the above-mentioned separation of zones, because through these I am able to distinguish yellow fever from other, certainly rare, liver diseases with necrosis of the intermediate zone."

Dr. Harald Seidelin (Y. F. Bulletin, Vol. III., No. 4, pp. 269-294, p. 271) has recently discussed this question in a paper on "The Histology of the Liver in Yellow Fever," in which he accepts Da Rocha Lima's description as that of a very common, but not constant, type of Yellow Fever liver. He finds a remarkable variation between the cases and also between different parts of the same organ.

Dr. Seidelin is of opinion that Da Rocha Lima has correctly described necrobiotic changes as the lesion of greatest importance in the Yellow Fever liver.

He gives (pp. 296-298, Plates VIII. and IX.), on Plate VIII. four figures from the same liver in which the types represented in Figs. 1 and 3 were common, and that of Fig. 2 much less common, and Fig. 4 distinctly rare.

The figures are thus described:—

"Fig. 1.—*Irregular type of necrobiosis.*—The necrobiotic areas are quite irregularly distributed, though slightly less marked in the peripheral zone than in the central and intermediate zones. Moderate fatty change. Slight cellular infiltration in some places where the necrosis is complete. Acid hæm-alum and eosin.

"Fig. 2.—*Rocha-Lima type of mid-zonal necrosis.*—The central and peripheral zones are well marked, consisting of well-preserved cells, with a few necrobiotic cells irregularly distributed amongst the others. In the intermediate zone conditions are reversed. Same stain. Otherwise similar to Fig. 1.

"Fig. 3.—*Peripheral type.*—The cells in the inner zone are fairly well preserved, but in the two outer zones they are either necrobiotic or the seat of extreme fatty change. With this low power the specimen shows considerable similarity to typical fatty infiltration. Hyperæmia of a hepatic vein type. Same stain.

"Fig. 4.—*Central type.*—The inner zone is severely affected, the middle zone slightly, and the outer zone hardly at all. Fatty change moderate. Van Gieson stain."

"Rocha-Lima has found that the necrotic changes are of a mid-zonal type, the middle zone being wider than the others and consisting almost entirely of necrotic cells together with erythrocytes and round cells; the inner zone is narrower than the outer one, and may consist only of a few cells; fatty change is marked in the outer and inner zones, but less marked in the necrotic area. This author emphasises that the phenomena are essentially the same in all cases, differing only in intensity; in the individual case the hepatic lesions are remarkably uniform throughout the organ. He declares that it is unjustified to speak of a general disorganisation of the liver parenchyma, although occasionally the trabecular structure may be interrupted in the necrotic areas.

"It is necessary to consider carefully this question of local distribution, because Rocha-Lima claims for the mid-zonal type of necrosis a considerable diagnostic importance. I have previously stated that, in my opinion, Rocha-Lima has described a very common, but not constant, type of yellow fever liver, and a careful revision of my old specimens, together with examination of sections from recent cases, has confirmed me in this view. Once having had the attention drawn to the Rocha-Lima type, I have been able to observe its presence in some cases in which I had not noticed it before, but there are others in which it is altogether absent or so rarely seen that it cannot by any means be spoken of as the type. Thus, considering my own results together with those of Carroll, Otto and Neumann, Marchoux and Simond, and Boyce, and comparing them with the description given by Rocha-Lima, I arrive at the conclusion that mid-zonal necrosis is common and often well marked, but that other types occur in a considerable number of cases, and that various types may be well marked in one and the same liver." (Y.F.B., Vol. III., No. 4, p. 271.)

Dr. Seidelin states (p. 291):—

Rocha-
, II. Da
2).
. Archiv.
h. u.
en Hyg.,
pp. 192-
Leipsig.
(1912).
andl.
tsch
ol. Ges.,
pp. 168-
(with dis-
on). Jena.
(1914).
Congr. of
., London,
. Sect.
pt. II.,
57-62,
lon.

"Rocha-Lima regards necrobiosis as the essential phenomenon, and is of opinion that a certain type of mid-zonal necrosis is characteristic of yellow fever. He admits already in his first papers (1912, 1 and 2)* that similar lesions may occur in other diseases, although not with exactly the same characters as in yellow fever.

"In the discussion following one of these papers (1912, 2), and in the later paper (1914), he declares that the mid-zonal necrosis is not pathognomonic, but of very rare occurrence in other infections: the few instances in which similar though not identical lesions have been demonstrated are cases of abdominal sepsis which could hardly be mistaken for yellow fever. The diagnostic importance of mid-zonal necrosis depends evidently on two factors: its common or constant occurrence in yellow fever and its non-occurrence in other diseases. With regard to the first point, I have already stated above that in my experience this type is quite common, but by no means constant, and I have quoted the descriptions by Carrol, Otto and Neumann, Marchoux and Simond, and Boyce, which do not conform to the Rocha-Lima type. To this evidence may be added that Turnbull (*vide infra*), in his two cases, has found a peripheral zone of comparatively well-preserved cells, but only in one of the cases a similar central one; in the other case the necrosis was equally marked in the central and intermediate zones. Stevenson's (1915) (*vide infra*) brief description, on the other hand, of the liver lesions in one case corresponds well to Rocha-Lima's type, so far as can be judged without further details."

No. 26,
, Vol. II,
581-594
93).

Dr. A. C. Stevenson, of the Wellcome Bureau of Scientific Research, was requested by the Commission to report on pathological material from a case diagnosed as Yellow Fever, which is given in detail in the Appendix to a Report by Dr. G. E. H. Le Fanu, on a "List of Fever cases investigated during the months of March and April, 1914."

The following is Dr. Stevenson's description of the microscopical appearances of a portion of the liver:—

"*Liver.*—Lobules not very defined. Liver cells around central vein show fatty change, as do also those on the outside of the lobule.

"In the zone between these is a markedly necrotic area in which cells having a markedly acidophil character appear; this zone is also much engorged with blood, which is not seen in the other zones. There is some small round cell infiltration of portal canals."

Hitherto, as Da Rocha Lima states, nearly all authors have laid stress on the importance of the fatty changes in the liver in Yellow

Fever, and rightly so, for such changes are undoubtedly present; but there is ample evidence proving that necrosis also occurs.

Specimens from two cases diagnosed as Yellow Fever were submitted by the Commission to Dr. Hubert M. Turnbull, Director of the Pathological Institute of the London Hospital, whose report and comments on the microscopical changes in the liver and other organs in these cases are contained in Vol. I. of the Reports on questions connected with the investigation of non-malarial fevers in West Africa, issued by the Commission:—

I. R., Vol. pp. 195–20 (p. 198), (p. 202), (p. 204).

"*Liver.*—The parenchyma is the seat of conspicuous degeneration. The hepatic cells are greatly swollen, and the capillaries appear to be completely occluded or are only recognised as narrow clefts. In only a few areas are red corpuscles seen in the capillaries. In paraffin sections stained in hæmatoxylin and eosin, there is usually a zone, two to four cells broad, immediately round the portal systems, in which the cells retain a polygonal shape, are for the most part free from vacuoles and have sharply stained nuclei. Internal to this there is a broad zone in which the protoplasm of the cells contain clear vacuoles of various sizes and is to a greater or less extent hyaline and deeply eosinophil. In the majority of the cells there are no nuclei; in others very faintly stained swollen nuclei can just be recognised. Other nuclei are shrunken and deformed; chromatolysis is, however, much the commonest expression of nuclear degeneration and necrosis. Where the cells can be differentiated they are rounded in shape; in this zone, however, it is usually impossible to differentiate individual cells or even cellular columns. In approximately the central half of the lobules the cells are to a large extent rounded and show a varying degree of vacuolation and hyaline, eosinophilic degeneration of their protoplasm, and chromatolysis, but these changes are much less severe, so that the cellular columns and individual cells can be differentiated. Within the columns of this zone there is a considerable amount of bright yellow bile-pigment.

"In sections stained with sudan the outer half of the lobules, with the exception of the narrow zone in the extreme periphery described above, is occupied by a large quantity of fatty substance. The fat does not form large, round droplets which evenly distend signet-shaped cells. The bulk of it is in form of medium-sized, deeply-stained droplets which lie in groups within degenerate cells. Fine intracellular granules are also present. Occasional large masses of round or irregular shape are extracellular, and obviously formed by the disintegration of cells. In the central half of the lobules there is much less fat, it is intracellular and in the form of small granules of 'dust.' In sections stained by Nile-blue-sulphate, less fat is demonstrated than in sudan; the smallest granules are not stained; the fat, almost without exception, gives the pink reaction of neutral fat. In preparations of cells crushed in water or in acetic acid and examined with a polarisator very small doubly refractile bodies are present."

The Kidneys.

The following is Dr. Turnbull's summary of the histological changes in the kidney of case 26 (p.202):—

"The *kidney* is icteric and shows extensive necrosis and parenchymatous degeneration. Necrosis of the first convoluted tubules is extreme and dominates the picture. Fatty degeneration is slight and is confined to the second convoluted tubules. Casts are present. There is no accumulation of iron pigment. There is no evidence of inflammatory action in the form of emigration of cells in the interstitial tissues."

Of the *kidney* in case L. 14 (p. 203) it is stated:—

"The changes in the *kidney* only differ in detail from those in Case L. 26. Necrosis of the parenchyma is much less marked and there is a corresponding increase in the expressions of degeneration. Thus fatty degeneration is much more marked in the second convoluted tubules, and is found also in the loops of heule and collecting tubules. Casts of albuminous, fibrinoid substances, especially a deeply eosinophil substance, are very numerous.

"As in Case 1, there is no evidence of inflammatory reaction, so that the term 'nephritis' is not justified."

The following is Dr. Turnbull's summary and analysis of the changes observed (p. 202):—

"*Summary and Analysis of Histological Abnormalities.*

"*Case* L. 26 (pp. 45 and 196).—The *liver* is the seat of a very severe parenchymatous degeneration and necrosis, in which an accumulation of fat is the most important feature and a hyaline alteration of the protoplasm is conspicuous. A narrow zone of hepatic case immediately round the portal systems is almost intact; the external half of the remainder of the lobule is much more severely affected than the central. The degenerate and necrosed cells compress and appear to constrict the capillaries. There is icterus and an accumulation of granules of iron pigment. There is no evidence of inflammatory reaction except an infiltration of the portal systems, which in its cytology resembles the infiltration found in the spleen.

"*Case* L. 14 (p. 219).—In the *liver* there is a slight portal fibrosis. The dense and sclerotic nature of the fibrous tissue excludes recent activity of the process; the fibrosis bears no constant relation to an infiltration which resembles that in Case L. 26, and which is only found in some of the portal systems. The slight portal fibrosis is evidently an accidental complication. The other histological changes differ from those in Case L. 26 in intensity alone. The degeneration and necrosis are greater, and the central portion of the lobules is as severely affected as the intermediate. There is a greater accumulation of iron pigment."

"*Significance of the difference in the two cases.*

"Death appears to have occurred at an earlier stage of the disease in Case L. 26, and the earlier onset of death was perhaps due to the rapid and extensive necrosis of the kidney. Thus in Case L. 14 the affection of the liver is severer, and when compared with Case L. 26 appears to have advanced towards the central veins. In the kidney degenerations are much more conspicuous, and there are greater accumulations of casts; the parenchymatous degeneration appears to have had longer time to develop. In the spleen the proliferation of endothelial cells is greater and the cells have become phagocytes.

"*Comparison with the Lesions of Yellow Fever described in the Literature.*

"The general features of the pathological changes in yellow fever, as described in the literature to which I have had access, are found in the two cases under discussion. These general features are:— Icterus. Severe parenchymatous degeneration and necrosis of the liver, in which fatty degeneration plays the most conspicuous *rôle*. A variable degree of parenchymatous degeneration and necrosis of the kidney, in which fatty degeneration may be very slight. Engorgement and hæmorrhage in the intestine, the hæmorrhage being greatest and usually very conspicuous in the stomach. A variable degree of inflammation and necrosis of the mucosa of the intestine. Engorgement of the pulp of the spleen. No constant nor characteristic change in the lung.

"Further, such details as are given in the descriptions of the histological changes are almost all found in the two cases under discussion. Thus, in the liver, Carroll (1905) describes a zone of cells round the portal systems in which degenerative changes are slight. He specially mentions a hyaline, deeply eosinophil, necrosis of the hepatic cells. Marchoux and Simond (1906) describe compression of the capillaries by swollen hepatic cells in cases in which death occurs between the fifth and tenth day. Carroll says that this compression is so constant and peculiar a feature that it can indeed be considered as characteristic of the disease. It may, however, be found in other diseases." (*Ibid*, pp. 204-205.)

It has possibly been too readily assumed from the presence in the urine of albumen and casts of the urinary tubules that there is a true nephritis in Yellow Fever. The evidence from two fatal cases showing the absence of such a condition is not of course conclusive, but it is sufficient to show that both albumen and casts of the renal tubes may be present in the urine in Yellow Fever, apart from inflammation of the kidneys. The point is also of importance in the differentiation of Malaria and Yellow Fever. In the section on that subject mention is made of the fact (*vide* p. 171) that in

America albuminuria has been frequently observed in severe cases of malignant tertian infection, and that nephritis follows in about 1·7 per cent. of such cases. This is relied on by those who seek to minimise the importance of albuminuria as a symptom of Yellow Fever, but we are not aware that nephritis has been observed as a sequela of Yellow Fever; indeed, it is remarkable how quickly the albumen and casts disappear from the urine in cases of that disease which recover. If the albuminuria and the casts were the expressions of a true nephritis, this would hardly be so, but if there is no inflammatory change it is easily understood.

Before a pathological lesion can be accepted as typical of a disease it must be shown to occur with such frequency that its absence in any given case is strongly presumptive against such a diagnosis. This obtains with regard to the lesions of Peyer's patches in Typhoid Fever, although it is true that cases have been reported in which they were normal yet such cases are extremely rare.

We do not think more can be claimed for Rocha Lima's mid-zonal necrosis than that it is a valuable and accurate observation, but the absence of that change in any case should not outweigh the evidence derived either from the clinical course of the disease, or from other post-mortem appearances; indeed, Rocha-Lima himself does not claim that it is invariably present.

SECTION XIII.

THE BLOOD IN YELLOW FEVER.

It is practically certain that the virus of Yellow Fever primarily infects the blood, and that, either therein or elsewhere in the body, it develops toxic products which circulate in the blood: The fact that by the inoculation of blood serum from a patient in the first three days of the illness it is possible to transmit the disease is sufficient proof of this.

...l, ...hilippine ...rnal of ...ence," ...l. I., No. 5, ...e, 1906.

Carrol, in the paper to which the reference is given, quotes Stitt as having observed a marked contrast between the condition of the blood in Dengue and Yellow Fever.

In Dengue he found a polymorphonuclear, as well as a general leucopenia, with a marked relative increase in the mononuclear leucocytes, whereas in the early stage of Yellow Fever the total leucocyte count was practically normal, and there was no diminution in the proportion ot polymorphonuclear leucocytes, this, on the contrary, was frequently found to be increased.

In the Report* prepared by Dr. Horn and Dr. Mayer, and issued by the Colonial Office in 1913, which deals with the epidemics in 1910 and 1911, a synopsis of the cases is given (pp. 88-91) and under "The Circulatory System, Blood and Ductless Glands" (p. 89), a table showing the differential leucocyte count in six cases (Nos. 41-46). This is here reproduced, with, for comparison, the average numbers in normal blood:—

Normal Percentage.		Case 41.	Case 42.		Case 43.	Case 44.	Case 45.		Case 46.
65 to 75 ...	Polymorphs ...	82·25	86·07	74·50	71·00	67·25	71·00	67·25	77·00
1 to 2	Large mononuclears ...	4·00	4·70	5·75	6·25	5·00	6·25	5·00	6·00
25 to 35 ...	Lymphocytes...	12·00	7·64	12·00	17·00	24·00	17·00	24·00	11·75
1 to 2	Eosinophiles ...	0·50	0·19	1·25	4·25	4·25	4·00	2·75	0·50
2 to 4	Transitionals...	1·25	0·76	6·25	1·50	0·25	1·50	0·25	4·75
$\frac{1}{4}$ to $\frac{1}{2}$	Mast. cells ...	—	0·38	0·25	—	1·75	—	1·75	—
		100·00	99·74	100·00	100·00	102·50	99·75	101·00	100·00
	Malaria Parasites ...	Nil.	Nil.	Nil.	Nil.	Nil.	Nil.	Nil.	Nil.
	Pigmented mononuclears	—	—	—	Nil.	Nil.	—	—	Nil.

Case 41.—A fatal case of Yellow Fever in a European, aet. 24. Death occurred on the fifth day of the illness, and on the day following admission to hospital. The count was therefore made on the fourth or fifth day of the disease.

Accra, May 23rd 1911.

Case 42.—A fatal case of Yellow Fever in a European, aet. 27. The first count was made on the fourth day of the disease; the second on the seventh day. Death occurred early on the eighth day.

Accra, May 23rd 1911.

Case 43.—A mild attack of Yellow Fever in a native labourer, age (?), who was at the time in a segregation camp, under observation as a contact. The blood count was made on the second or possibly on the third day of the disease.

Accra, May 23rd 1911.

* See footnote, p. 25.

Case 44.—A mild attack in a native labourer, aet. about 30 years, who was also in the segregation camp under observation as a contact. The blood count was made on the second day of the disease.

Case 45.—The patient was a native clerk, aet. about 40 years. Recovery took place after an illness lasting 12 days. The first blood count was taken on the fourth day of the disease, the second on the seventh day.

Case 46.—A fatal case in a European, aet. 35 years. Death occurred on the fifth day of the disease. The blood count was probably taken on the second or third day.

The following blood counts are from fatal cases recorded by Dr. T. M. Russell Leonard in a report on "Certain Outbreaks of Yellow Fever in Lagos, 1913, and January and February, 1914":—

Case.	E—European. N—Native.	Age.	Day of Death.	Day of Count.	Result of Blood Examination.
No. 1. L 14 ...	E	28	5th	3rd	No malaria parasites present Leucopenia present. Polymorphonuclear, 71%. Mononuclear, 20%. Lymphocytes, 4%. Eosinophil, 5%. Hæmoglobin, 85%. Blood pressure, 125
No. 7. L 37 ...	E	34	5th	2nd	No malaria parasites present. Pigmented leucocytes present. Polymorphonuclear, 78%. Mononuclear, 7%. Lymphocytes, 13%. Eosinophil, 2%. Leucopenia present.
No. 8. L 38 ...	Syrian	40	5th	2nd	No malaria parasites present. Pigmented leucocytes present. Polymorphonuclear, 78·7%. Lymphocytes, 12%. Mononuclear, 8·3%. Eosinophil 1%
No. 11. L. 41 ...	Syrian	35	5th	2nd	No malaria parasites present. Pigmented leucocytes present. Polymorphonuclear, 76%. Mononuclear, 7%. Lymphocytes, 13%. Eosinophil, 4%.

The following cases of a milder type ending in recovery occurred in contacts under observation:—

Case.	E—European. N—Native.	Age.	Day of Death.	Day of Count.	Result of Blood Examination.
No. 9. L 39 ...	Syrian	24	—	2nd	No malaria parasites were found. Pigmented leucocytes. Polymorphonuclear, 75·5% Mononuclear, 6%. Lymphocytes, 15%. Eosinophils, 3·5%.
No. 14. L 44 ...	E	30	—	—	No malaria parasites present. Differential count : Polymorphonuclear, 80%. Mononuclear, 2·5%. Lymphocytes, 17%. Eosinophil, 0·5%.
No. 19. L 52 ...	N	20	—	2nd	No malaria parasites present. Pigmented lencocytes present. Leucopenia present. Polymorphonuclear, 68·5%. Lymphocytes, 18·5%. Mononuclear, 8·5%. Eosinophil, 0·3%. Transitionals, 4·2%.

Dr. J. M. O'Brien visited Guayaquil, Ecuador, in October, 1913, with a view to study Yellow Fever in an endemic area. In a report* on his visit furnished to the Commission, he gives (p. 320) the results of his microscopical examinations of the blood in the Yellow Fever cases which he observed there:— I.R., Vol I pp. 317-35

"Differential leucocyte counts present the following points of interest:—

"The percentage of polymorphonuclears is nearly always high.

"The number of large mononuclears is generally normal.

"The lymphocytes sometimes diminish almost to disappearing point, but, on the other hand, in some well-defined cases of yellow fever, maintain their percentage normally high.

"Eosinophils are frequently absent, but the same may be said of natives of Ecuador in other diseases.

"The percentage of transitionals varies between the usual limits of my counts. Mast cells are commonly present. The differential counts in general suggest an increase in the percentage of polymorphonuclears, rather than a decrease in the other elements.

* NOTE.—This report is also published in the "Annals of Tropical Medicine and Parasitology," Liverpool, December, 1914, Vol. VIII., pp. 369-378, with plate, but without the appendix

"With regard to the occasional very low percentage of lymphocytes, judging from the small number of slides I have been able to examine, I think that a low lymphocyte count is normal to the people of this country.

"As convalescence progresses the percentages adjust themselves to the normal."

Dr. Seidelin, in a review of Dr. O'Brien's results, writes as follows:— I., 3–361.

"These results differ from those obtained by other recent observers, but correspond fairly well to the leucocyte counts given by Arevedo and Conto."

Dr. Seidelin analyses the 47 differential counts contained in the Appendix to Dr. O'Brien's paper, and finds that (p. 359):—

"In thirty the percentage of polymorphonuclear cells is above 70, whilst in three it is between 65 and 70, and in fourteen below 65. Amongst the latter we find two in which the percentage is 44 and four in which it lies between 45 and 55. On the other hand, the percentage of mononuclears, as distinct from lymphocytes, and therefore presumably 'large mononuclears,' is given as 10 or higher in twenty-three cases, and in several other cases it is close to 10; in some cases the percentages are as high as 24·3, 25·3 and 28·6.

"This is very far from normal conditions. According to these figures, O'Brien's results do not differ very materially from those obtained by the reviewer in Yucatan. Some of the mononuclear percentages are probably the highest hitherto recorded."

A Change in the Polymorphonuclears.

'ol. I., 7–352. Dr. O'Brien describes (p. 321) a change in the polymorphonuclears, which he thinks may prove to be of diagnostic value. He believes that in a very large proportion of Yellow Fever cases these cells are acutely degenerated and in a wholesale manner:—

"In a typical case, about the third day of the fever, some half of the polymorphonuclears lose the brown, stippled, staining reaction which their protoplasm has towards giemsa; by the fourth day all have lost this colouring; only faint dots may be seen in the cytoplasm, in others the cytoplasm is obviously unstained and hardly discernible. The nucleus in this stage remains normal.

"In the next stage the protoplasm edge looks torn and ragged, the nucleus becomes splayed out and lightly stained; without having seen the various stages of the transformation, it would be difficult to recognise the cell.

"Later, the protoplasm contracts, assumes a rounded form and takes on a light pink colour. The nucleus is round and small—its stain becomes intense.

"In the most advanced stage observed the nucleus is round, with perhaps one or two drop-shaped fragments of nuclear matter near it. The cytoplasm is circular, and about twice the size of a red corpuscle. It has a pinkish stain. More than anything else it suggests in shape a small *amœbacol.* This form is scarcely scattered in the slides."

Dr. Seidelin, in the review just mentioned, expresses a doubt whether the cells shown in the plate,* which accompanies Dr. O'Brien's paper, except a very few, are really polymorphonuclear leucocytes.

*"Ann. Trop. Med Paras." Liverpool, December, 1914, Vol. VIII., pp. 369-37

THE HÆMOGLOBIN IN YELLOW FEVER.

The following account of the condition of the blood in Yellow Fever is from the "Manual of Tropical Medicine" by Castellani and Chalmers:—

"*The Blood.*—There is no marked alteration in the numbers or appearance of the erythrocytes, even in fatal cases. A few normoblasts are said to be present at times. On the other hand, there is a decided loss of hæmoglobin, though this is rarely much reduced in the first three or four days; and hæmoglobinæmia is said to occur in fatal cases before death. But this does not appear to coincide with the fall of specific gravity, which may be present without loss of hæmoglobin. The leucocytes do not appear to be distinctly increased in numbers, varying from 3,200 to 20,000 per cubic millimetre, the increase, when present, being largely caused by polymorphonuclear leucocytes. The coagulation of the blood is diminished, and ammonæmia is thought to be present in bad cases."

Castellani & Chalmers, "Manual of Tropical Medicine," 2nd Ed., p. 1,009.

Carrol writes as follows (1):—

"Guiteras (2) * * * * * * lays special stress upon the value of the estimation of hæmoglobin, the percentage of which in yellow fever is rarely below 90 in the first three, four or five days. He states that if the percentage is found to be below 80 in the first few days in a case of yellow fever some complication will always be found or the patient will have previously suffered from malaria."

(1) Osler & McCrae, "System of Medicine," Art., "Yellow Fever" by James Carroll, M.D. Vol. p. 753.

(2) "Medical Age," Detroit, Vol. XXIV. No. 6, March 25, 1906.

It may, however, be pointed out that on the West Coast of Africa it is very unusual indeed to find in a European in a normal state of health for that region such a high percentage of hæmoglobin as 90 per cent. or even 80 per cent.

The reason for this is, no doubt, as Guiteras suggests, that they have previously suffered from Malaria, but it follows that as an aid to diagnosis in Yellow Fever the observation is of restricted value in that part of the world. It might, however, be useful in the case of a European who had recently arrived on the Coast.

SECTION XIV.

MOSQUITOES.

In December, 1909, the Advisory Medical and Sanitary Committee for Tropical Africa passed the following resolution:—"The Committee recommend that the attention of Governors should be drawn to the necessity of its being laid down as a *sine quâ non* that at least a part of an officer's quarters be protected against mosquitoes; and that the Secretary of State should express a strong opinion that where mosquito protection is afforded, it should be used"; and in accordance with their recommendation a report was called for, by the Secretary of State, from the Governors of the East and West African Dependencies on the subject of rendering mosquito-proof at least a part of an officer's quarters.

In October, 1910, following on the outbreaks in that year of Yellow Fever in Freetown, Seccondee and elsewhere, a despatch was sent to the Governors of the British Colonies and Protectorates in West Africa, asking for information as to the progress made during the preceding six months in the elimination of the *Stegomyia fasciata* from the various towns concerned.

In Northern Nigeria the native Emirs manifested great interest in the matter, and the Emir of Kano issued a Proclamation, of which the following is a translation. It is worthy of being placed on record:—

"From the Emir of Kano Abbas to all the People of Kano.

"(Translation from the Arabic.)

"Know that my command is as follows:—

"Whereas we have been informed by the Governor's physician of four important matters; every one must take notice of these matters.

"First of all, the sick infect the healthy, so that they become sick in turn.

"The mosquito sucks the blood of the sick man, and then goes to the healthy and bites him and infuses the blood of the sick into the healthy. The blood of the sick infects the blood of the healthy, and in the most cases the healthy becomes sick by the power of God and His will, since the affairs of the world are regulated by cause and effect. Truly the world is subject to these laws.

"Therefore we should take measures to reduce the number of mosquitoes and kill them off. The mosquito, as is known, breeds in wells and pits, and old pots, and earth holes; we should not make a pit near houses. Whoever has a pit or hole or old well near his house, let him fill it up.

"Secondly, we are informed that the common fly bites lepers, and then bites the healthy, and then leprosy is conveyed to the healthy by the power of God and His will, so that the healthy man becomes a leper.

"Therefore, we must take steps to reduce the flies. The fly, as is known, breeds in middens and refuse heaps and garbage and filth and places where blood is collected, like shambles.

"We must get the people to clean up and bury all refuse of this sort.

"Every butcher must cover the blood of oxen and sheep, and must slaughter far away from markets, and wash the meat, and clear the blood away, and bring the clean meat to the market to avoid attracting many flies.

"Thirdly, as regards venereal disease—many women here are diseased. If they cohabit with the healthy, the healthy become infected.

"I command all my alkalis to punish severely any person who conveys infection to another, either man or woman.

"Fourthly, concerning the wells, which, when the water is infected, convey dysentery and guinea-worm.

"We order that all owners of wells shall surround the mouth of the well with a parapet, to prevent infection being conveyed into the well and the well being spoilt.

"Nor should the excrement of cattle be allowed to get into wells, for this pollutes the wells.

"But, you are informed, if water is boiled, that kills the infection in the water.

"Those who have sense and respect their health should attend to this advice and boil drinking water.

"You, my brothers, do not forget the words of the Prophet in the Hadith's, which are full of learning and wisdom. He says. 'All that God wills for man has its cause writ plain.' From God we obtain help and on Him do we rely. There is no strength or help save in God Most High.

"PEACE."

The Commission are indebted to the Imperial Bureau of Entomology for information as to the distribution of mosquitoes in West Africa, as shown by records in the possession of the Bureau and by material preserved in the British Museum.

From this it appears that *S. fasciata* is present in nearly all the places from which cases of Yellow Fever have been reported.

Frequent reference has been made in the course of this Report to the Abeokuta case (*vide* p. 54).

Dr. E. J. Wyler, who reported on that case, gives the following description of the

Vol. I., "*Conditions as regards* Stegomyia *in Abeokuta and other places visited by patient, especially near residence of, and places frequented by, patient.*

"The conditions throughout Abeokuta are very favourable to breeding of *Stegomyia*. Water is obtained from wells by the natives (only those living in that part of the town which is nearest the river use river water), and is carried and stored in uncovered earthenware pots varying in capacity from one to eight gallons. (The manufacture of these pots is an important local industry.) Practically every compound contains large numbers of these vessels; in one selected at random in which ten persons lived there were thirty-three.

"Some of these pots are sunk in the ground (often nearly to the brim) and are therefore never completely emptied. Moreover all wells (except three) are privately owned, and a charge, varying with season, is made for water. Hence it is to the financial interest of the native to economise water and to empty his water pot as slowly as possible. In one compound, for example, there were twelve pots, eleven of which contained larvæ. In three compounds chosen at random there were fifty-two pots; thirty-five of these contained larvæ, largely *Stegomyia*, nine were dry, and eight contained water without larvæ. These compounds were within 200 yards of the patient's house.

"I have examined forty compounds in widely separated parts of the town and have found larvæ in all of them without exception. *Stegomyia fasciata* are present in considerable numbers, and form a large proportion of all larvæ. This I have ascertained by actual hatching out. I have examined a number of water-tanks (filled by rain from the roof) attached to European dwellings, and found larvæ in most of them (88 per cent.).

"In most cases no serious attempt at mosquito proofing has been made. In others the proofing has been allowed to fall into disrepair. In the deceased's house, which stands in a thickly populated part of the town and is surrounded by native dwellings, the nearest European house being over half-a-mile distant, I found a cooler (a native earthenware vessel containing water, which, by evaporation of water through its walls, cools syphons, &c., immersed therein) in which *Stegomyia* larvæ were numerous. This was an experience which I repeated in other European houses.

"These water pots, whether in the houses of careless Europeans or in native compounds and houses, are the chief source of *Stegomyia* breeding during the dry season. The tins, broken bottles, and vessels of all kinds which are thrown down at random and apparently never cleared away doubtless form ideal breeding places in the wet season, lying free from disturbance among the rank grass and bush that abounds throughout the town.

"There had been very little rain in Abeokuta up to the time of my investigations there, and I did not find larvæ elsewhere than in the earthenware pots mentioned, in water-butts, and in one tin in which water had been placed.

"Except in some of the better class native houses there are no latrines for natives in this town of 51,255 inhabitants (official census, 1911), the patches of uncleared bush and grass being used for this purpose.

"One such patch, with the usual accretion of tins, bottles, &c., I found situated within a few *feet* of the patient's house.

"The sanitary conditions generally which obtain in Abeokuta may, without over-statement, be described as deplorable, and as being calculated to foster not only yellow fever, but also enteric disease and (as already been demonstrated) small-pox.

"I have elsewhere mentioned that the native houses, though roofed with corrugated iron, are almost invariably devoid of gutters, so that this source of water-stagnation is not significant. I examined seventeen wells and nine ponds in widely distant parts of the town, but did not find *Stegomyia* larvae in any of them. The water was very low at the time in consequence of the retardation of the rains."

It should be pointed out that Abeokuta is situated in the native State of Egba, and that the responsibility for the insanitary conditions described above rested with the native government of that State. It must not be concluded that no efforts have been made to remedy these conditions during the period which has elapsed since the issue of that Report.

On August 22nd, 1913, a patient, whose case is described on p. 57 of this Report, was admitted to Lagos Hospital for observation, and the diagnosis of Yellow Fever was made on the following day. He had been staying for one month at Ogbomosho, and had travelled to Lagos *viâ* Oyo, Fiditi and Ibandan, and thence by rail to Lagos. He was removed from the train at Lagos as he was found during the routine examination of passengers to be suffering from pyrexia (103° F.).

Dr. E. J. Wyler proceeded to Ogbomosho, and made the following Report as to the conditions:—

, Vol. I., 31-33.

"*Conditions as regards* Stegomyia *breeding in Ogbomosho and other places visited by patient, and near his residence.*

"I found from actual breeding out of larvæ that *Stegomyia fasciata* is present in Ogbomosho, Oyo, Fiditi, and Ibadan.

"The conditions in all these towns for *Stegomyia* breeding are favourable, there being numerous water-pots in the native compounds. Larvæ are abundant.

"*S. fasciata* larvæ were numerous in the patient's compound at Ogbomosho."

Dr. Wyler discusses the question as to the place where this patient acquired his infection in the following paragraph of the Report:—

"*Conclusions.*

"I conclude that the patient must have acquired his infection either in Ogbomosho or in Oyo. He *might* have acquired it at Fiditi; but in that case the incubation period must have been fifty-four hours or less. It is scarcely possible that he became infected in Ibadan, since the number of hours between his arrival in that town and his detention at Lagos on the following afternoon would connote an incubation period of (at the most) thirty hours, and the number of hours between sunset on the day of his arrival in Ibadan and the time of his detention in Lagos would imply an even shorter incubation period (twenty-two hours). In spite of the fact, however, that infective *Stegomyia* bite only after sunset, this latter period of twenty-two hours seems here hardly to be of significance, for native houses are, as a rule, exceedingly dark, the interiors being in very many instances maintained in such a state of perpetual night that persons frequenting them would be liable to become infected at any period of the twenty-four hours.

"These conclusions as to the locality in which the patient was infected are based on the supposition that the date of his admission to hospital coincided with the first day of his illness. When I questioned him in hospital he denied having any subjective symptoms, or having experienced any in the past few days, though I understand that when previously interrogated by the Resident Medical Officer he gave the impression that he was, on admission, in the fifth day of the disease. In this latter case he must have acquired the disease in Ogbomosho. Statements of native patients regarding their health are, of course, frequently of doubtful value. Since in none of the towns visited by the patient within a month of the onset of his illness have there been any suspicious European cases, it appears to be clear that (excluding a hypothetical animal source of infection) the patient acquired the disease from another native.

"E. J. W.

"*6th September, 1913.*"

In May and June, 1913, there was an outbreak of Yellow Fever at Warri (*vide* p. 60) when two Europeans engaged in a factory (store) contracted the disease, one of whom died.

The following extracts are from Dr. E. J. Wyler's Report on the

"*Conditions as regards* Stegomyia *Breeding at Warri, especially near residence of and places frequented by the patients.* I.R., Vol. pp. 70-72.

"I inspected a large proportion of the compounds of European officials, native officials, and the general native population, and found them very free from breeding places.

"This was also the case in regard to the premises of the mercantile firms, all of which I inspected. Only once did I find larvæ in Warri during my inquiry: in one of the trader's compounds on the river bank. They were in the zinc lining of a packing-case that was in use as a receptacle for rubbish.

"I inspected sixty-three native dwellings; eleven canoes (not in use); thirty-three water-tanks (in five the gauze was defective); twelve rain gutters; and eleven receptacles for water, such as metal pots, barrels, &c., all taken at random. There were no larvæ in any of them. The wells were covered in with one exception, and in this also I failed to find larvæ.

"There are two villages of moderate size within approximately half-a-mile of Warri. I inspected thirty-six of the houses and found larvæ in none, in spite of the fact that some water pots raised on wooden tripods in the streets in connexion with fetish worship were swarming with them. These villages are subject to frequent visits by the Sanitary Inspector.

"The water supply in Warri for both Europeans (rain-water tanks) and natives (mainly well-water) is, I am informed, adequate, so that there is no necessity for undue economy and protracted storage.

"The occurrence of cases of yellow fever would naturally have the effect of greatly stimulating anti-mosquito measures, so that the conditions as I found them some time afterwards probably afford no adequate indication of the state of affairs at the time. I therefore quote the following remarks from a report made in June by the Acting Sanitary Officer :—

"'Distribution of *Stegomyia.* They are found more or less all over the station, but were undoubtedly very much more numerous along the river front in the European traders' compounds than anywhere else. In some of these, *Stegomyia* larvæ were found in large numbers in roof gutters, packing-cases, barrels, tins, &c., and * * *'s compound had by far the largest number of breeding places. There was a large collection of empty packing-cases piled up behind * * *'s shop, and the rains had caused the wood to swell so much that the lower tiers were capable of containing six or more inches of water. *Stegomyia* larvæ were found in these in large numbers.

"'Two or three days after the removal of this breeding place, the shop, which had been infested with mosquitoes, was comparatively free from them. In the Government Rest House, which is situate next to * * *'s compound and to leeward of it, there were also many mosquitoes, with a fair number of *Stegomyia* amongst them, which had doubtless come from Messrs. * * *'s compound.*

"'The compounds of the European officials, native clerks, and general native population were remarkably free from breeding places. In the pond and numerous water-holes on the golf course there were enormous numbers of mosquito-larvæ; considerable numbers were collected and hatched out but none proved to be *Stegomyia*. Those hatched out were species of *Culex* and *Pyretophorus*.'†

"I was informed by the Agent of a trading company that the number of mosquitoes, especially during the first half of the year, appeared to be much in excess of previous experience.

"On inspecting their premises I observed a number of canoes (eleven) moored at their wharf (see Plan I.). These canoes were laden for the most part with native food-stuffs. I was informed that there is a constant succession of craft which make this wharf their stopping place. They come from widely separated parts of the Niger Delta, and frequently remain alongside overnight. I was unable to discover any larvæ in the water which they nearly all contained to a greater or less extent, probably because canoes in use have frequently to be baled out. (In canoes which are not in use larvæ may often be found.) The presence of infected natives in such canoes would, however, constitute a perpetual danger to the European inhabitants of the firm's compound.

"The firm's agent informed me that canoes from Burutu (*vide* Section II.) usually go to Ogbe Ijoh (New Warri) and do not stop at their wharf, but that natives disembark from the bi-weekly launch from Foreados and Burutu opposite their premises, which often remains moored to the wharf until the following day. The facilities, therefore, for the transport of infection direct from Burutu and Forcados, where cases in natives were occurring at the time of the Warri outbreak (Section II.) were considerable. It will be seen also (Section II., paragraphs VI. and VII.) that launches and steamers which moor alongside the wharves may play no small part in the reinforcement of the supply of *Stegomyia* mosquitoes in Warri.

"* This Rest House has since been rendered mosquito-proof.—E.J.W."

"† In view of the fact that Dr. Laurie, the Junior Sanitary Officer, had found *Stegomyia* breeding in pools at Forcados—Section II.—I carefully investigated the possibility of similar conditions existing at Warri. I failed, however, to find larvæ in any pools, or in swamp near the town. The pools mentioned above by the Acting Sanitary Officer as existing on the golf course had dried up at the time of my visit.—E.J.W."

"The following are the mosquito indices (all varieties) for the years 1912 and 1913, based on the observations of Native Sanitary Inspectors :—

		"1912.	1913.
"Quarter ending 31st March	...	0·2	0·23
,, ,, 30th June	...	0·48	0·51
,, ,, 30th September	...	0·45	0·36
,, ,, 31st December	...	0·23	—"

In Dr. E. J. Wyler's "Fourth Report on Yellow Fever in Ships and in the Central Province," the following were the

"*Conditions as regard* Stegomyia *Breeding in Forcados and Burutu.* I.R Vol. pp. 42–19 pp. 151–1!

"*Stegomyia fasciata* is present at both Foreados and Burutu.

"The native houses in those towns are disposed on a definite plan.

"They stand, for the most part, in rows, are therefore easily inspected, and only a small proportion of them have compounds (inclosures), in which, in other towns, one so frequently finds colleetions of standing water and agglomerations of garbage. It is to be remarked, however, that in some parts of Foreados, notably in the area where Cases 22, 33, 36, 38, 41 occurred, the sanitary conditions were deplorable, and due entirely, I was informed, to the want of financial means to carry out some most essential and even elementary improvements. I inspected both Forcados and Burutu, in which the conditions as regards *Stegomyia* breeding are similar, and the following statistics represent the sum of my observations in both places, made before any exceptional anti-mosquito measures had been taken.

"Out of 115 houses taken at random in different parts of the towns, including those in which the cases described occurred, no water at all was found in 32, while in four larvæ were found These larvæ, on being hatched out, proved to be *Stegomyia fasciata.*

"My inspection, it should be remarked, was made at the termination of the rainy season, when the water supply is sufficient and there is no temptation to store it unduly inside the houses. The conditions which obtain in the dry season may possibly be less favourable, for, at that period of the year, I am informed, there is often a considerable shortage of water, which has then to be brought a long distance by river and economized as much as possible. This shortage, I am further informed, is due to the inadequate supply of rain-water tanks. I learned from the Medical Officer that the outbreak of four cases (Nos. 10, 11, 12, 15) in one house at Burutu was ascribable to the breeding of large numbers of *S. fasciata* in some barrels of water in the compound which had been overlooked by the Sanitary Inspector.

"Out of fifteen wells I found that six were safely screened; in one the mosquito gauze was in disrepair; in one (upon private ground) no attempt at screening had been made, in one (upon Government property) *Stegomyia* larvæ had been found according to the Sanitary Inspector. This well was unscreened and had since been oiled.

"I examined 37 rain-water tanks. Of these 29 were effectively screened. In eight the gauze was defective. Out of 34 barrels used for the storage of water, 15 were effectively screened, there was a defect in the gauze in 11, whilst 8 were open.

"In seven roof-gutters there was some standing water. In none of the wells, tanks, barrels, or roof-gutters, whether screened or not, did I find any larvæ whatever. The mosquito-index in Foreados, based on the observations of native sanitary inspectors in April, May, and June, 1913 (wet months), was 0·61, 0·46, 0·55, respectively.

"In December, 1912, and January and February, 1913 (dry months), it was 0·27, 0·61, 1·06, respectively.

"I inspected both the native villages, the nearest of which, as already stated, is about one furlong from a European residence (non-official).

"These villages are situated amidst unreclaimed swamp. The huts, which, even in the dry season are practically surrounded by water, are built of reeds and are raised, some upon piles, others upon platforms of earth. They are connected with one another and with the town by raised paths which slope down to the water on either side through a zone of black mud. The picture presented is that of a diminutive, primitive, and infinitely hideous and squalid Venice. The water is, for the most part, tidal, and I found no larvæ therein, but there are numerous ponds and pools where earth has been excavated to form platforms for houses. These are only reached by high tides, and in some (but in only one of the villages) I found an abundance of mosquito larvæ.

"Dr. Laurie, the Junior Sanitary Officer, had, I was informed, found some of these larvæ to be *Stegomyia fasciata*, but though I collected and bred out a large number, none of them proved to belong to this species. His observation is, of course, of the highest importance as indicating a probable source of supply of this insect to Forcados port.

"I obtained some of the water from the pond in question for analysis by the Government chemist, Mr. Ralston, in order that the degree of its salinity might be ascertained. He reported that the chlorides present were equivalent to 4·74 per cent. of common salt, and he informed me that, in a series of experiments carried out by him in 1904, he found that in water containing under 1 per cent. common salt mosquito larvæ developed freely.

"In consequence of the vigorous house inspection that had taken place in these villages, and the strict injunctions issued to the inhabitants concerning water storage prior to my visit, further examination would not have yielded any useful results.

"Twenty houses, taken at random, contained no larvæ; indeed, in a considerable proportion of these no water whatever was stored.

"From consideration of the foregoing facts it would appear that the river craft, and perhaps also, as regards Forcados, the native villages, constitute the principal source of supply of *S. fasciata* in

Forcados and Burutu.* As is well known, the insect breeds freely in the bilge water of river boats. Shallow, transverse steel girders, projecting a variable distance inwards from the inner surface, divide the hulls into compartments that form ideal pools for *Stegomyia* propagation. In the transomes and chain-lockers these pools are particularly difficult of access.

"I inspected one 'stern-wheeler' and two launches, and in all three *Stegomyia* were numerous.

"It may here be remarked that cases 6, 21, 35, were employed on river craft. This would necessitate their frequent presence on board at night. Case 31, though employed on ship-board, was probably infected ashore."

In a Report entitled "Notes on a visit to Sherbro District," by Drs. J. M. Dalziel and W. B. Johnson, it appears that at the date of the visit, January 27th to February 12th, 1913, no rain had fallen for two months, and that as a consequence no *Stegomyia* larvæ were found in the bottles, tins, etc., which were utilised for the purpose of filling up the numerous burrow-pits and hollows everywhere met with:— I.R., Vol. pp, 527-5[illegible]

"At the present season mosquitoes are not a pest—a few Europeans even dispense with the mosquito-net at this time of year—but one has no difficulty in observing a few every evening. *During the rains everyone admits that they are abundant*, but there is no record of the species found or of which are the most prevalent. Small domestic receptacles being so abundant and carelessly disposed of, one naturally suspects the *Stegomyia* to be predominant, *and this is vouched for by previous medical officers who have worked at Bonthe. Our search in the present month of February, however, has not revealed a single specimen of* Stegomyia." p. 529.

"Turning now to the search for mosquitoes and larvæ in Bonthe, the chief fact to record is the apparent absence at the present season of *Stegomyia*. One cannot, however, lay stress on this, and we may point to a similar absence of *Anophelines*, although there is no lack of enlarged spleens, and malaria parasites were readily found in a considerable proportion of the blood examinations. Both types are probably abundant in Bonthe during the rains, but there is no record of a mosquito survey, and one cannot therefore tell which are actually the prevalent species.

"A complete house-to-house inspection of the whole town was not made, but each day a number of compounds and lots were gone over in all the different quarters, and thus a total of 82 came under

---

"* Mosquitoes have also been found to breed in the numerous tortuous burrows of crabs. These may perhaps be a not inconsiderable source of *Stegomyia*, especially in the dry season, when they are not, as in the wet season, subject to constant flushing. The level of the subsoil water at Forcados, to which the burrows may extend, is within one or two feet of the surface.—E.J W."

examination. Mosquito larvæ were found five times—once in a surface well or uncovered water-hole which had fallen into disuse, twice in shallow wells with ill-fitting covers, once in a barrel, and once in domestic utensils (one bottle, and one earthen jar).

"All the larvæ found were other than *Stegomyia.* These figures give a larva index of 6 per cent. (wells being included). The available figures for the larva index taken on previous occasions are given below, but it is to be noted that the earlier figures at least exclude wells:—

"LARVA INDEX.

	"Bonthe.	York Island.
"March, 1911	12%	—
"May, 1911	11·8%	3·3%
"August, 1912	7%	—
"December, 1912	5%	—
"March, 1913 (quarter) ...	—	—
"June, 1913 ,, ...	3%	2%

"No figures are given for the larva index during the rains subsequent to June, 1913, but the sanitary gang appear to have become slack in their duties and lacked close supervision. The number of summonses for all breaches of sanitary laws fell suddenly from 40 in July to 6 in August and zero in September and October, so that it is more than probable that domestic mosquitoes again multiplied, and all residents admit that they were very numerous a few months ago.

"As stated above, our search failed to reveal a single *Stegomyia* larva, yet on looking over past sanitary reports we are confronted with the following, which is also a dry season record:—

> "'On May 1st, 1911, Dr. Burrows, Medical Officer of Health, Sherbro, reported on a '*Stegomyia* census' of 105 houses (75 in Bonthe and 30 in York Island). The resulting figures were:—
>
> "'Percentage of 'Larvæ Houses' in Bonthe—11·8
> ,, ,, ,, ,, York Island—3·3.'

"The larvæ found were stated in every case to be *Stegomyia,* and in one case mixed with *Anopheles* larvæ. The prevailing weather was dry, but Dr. Burrows remarks: 'An increase of 75 per cent. might safely be anticipated during the rains, as I found *Stegomyia* larvæ (which bred true) in every house I inspected in Bonthe in August last year (1910).' In the following year, in the height of the rains (August, 1912), Dr. Orpen recorded a larva index of only 7 per cent., and in his report comments on the unexpected difference between this figure and that predicted above. His house-to-house inspection was very carefully and completely worked out, and he suggests as possible explanations of the reduction of larvæ to such a low figure in the wet season, the following:—

> "(1) Heavy rainfall (36·6 inches) during the said month, perhaps 'flushing and keeping flushed the various articles capable of holding water.'

"(2) A vigorous campaign during the previous week against dirty compounds, resulting in a series of summonses.

"(3) The vigilance of the occupants (as a result of the sanitary campaign and its penalties), who immediately bustle about and empty every tub, barrel, pot, etc., leaving the yard still wet, when the cry 'Doctor do come' is raised.

"It is probable that the second of the above suggestions holds the key to the solution, and that in Bonthe, as in Freetown and everywhere else, the strict enforcement of regulations for domestic sanitation and a well-maintained supervision are essential, and are generally effective in reducing domestic-breeding mosquitoes to a proportion which probably ceases to be dangerous.

"It may be added that in Sherbro, as in Freetown and elsewhere in Sierra Leone, a common hedge plant is a variety of *Dracæna*, which retains water in the axils of the leaves. In Freetown a few months ago *Stegomyia* larvæ were found in this situation in many compound fences, and in Bonthe the plant has been proved to be a prolific source of mosquitoes during the rains."

"*No specimen of* Stegomyia *or of any* Anopheline *species was found, either adult or larvæ, in any compound.*" 533, p. 53

Two visits were made to York Island, which is near Sherbro, and consists of a smaller settlement on another reach of the branching creeks.

Here "*Again no* Stegomyia *were found, either larvæ or adult.*"

The following also occurs in the same Report, and is headed "Notes on a visit to Yonni on Sherbro Island":—

"Mosquitoes swarm in the village at night, but of 65 specimens which I (W. B. J.) caught during an hour or so in my house in the evening, 64 were *Mansonioides uniformis* and one was *Culex consimilis*. The former is a mangrove-breeding mosquito; and the absence of *Stegomyia* larvæ in the village shows that *in the dry season no disease depending upon that mosquito could occur.*"

These statements, which we have italicised, are important and suggestive.

It has perhaps been too readily assumed that because *Stegomyia* have been found in a certain place at a certain season of the year, whether during the rains or the dry season, they are therefore always present during that season in every year.

It appears that this is certainly not the case at Bonthe, possibly, therefore, not so elsewhere.

If, for the sake of illustration, we assume that Bonthe had been an endemic focus of Yellow Fever from a certain date up to

February, 1913, it is possible that in that year it would have ceased to be so owing to the complete absence of the carrier in any form, assuming that the absence lasted for a sufficiently long period.

It may therefore be that one of the causes of the disappearance of the disease from any place where its presence has been observed, either in a sporadic or epidemic form, is due to some exceptional condition leading to the complete absence of the *Stegomyia* from that place.

We know that without the carrier the disease cannot continue to exist, and that where this absence has been the result of human efforts the disease has disappeared; it is, therefore, a legitimate conclusion that the same result must follow where Nature and not man has been the agent at work.

In July, 1914, the Commission entrusted to Mr. A. W. Bacot, F.E.S., of the Lister Institute, whose work on the bionomics of the rat flea, in connection with Plague, is well known, a research at Sierra Leone on the life history of the *Stegomyia fasciata*, and the results are embodied in an admirable Report, which will be found in the third volume of the Investigators' Reports. The conclusions at which Mr. Bacot arrived are thus stated:—

"SUMMARY OF CONCLUSIONS.

"(1) Adult mosquitoes are scarce within the central area of Freetown, but the larvæ of *Stegomyia fasciata* are found in greater numbers than those of other varieties within the town.

"*Eggs.*

"(2) The dark spindle-shaped eggs of *S. fasciata* vary so considerably in shape and size, that it is not practical to distinguish them from the other species of the genus, which are distinct from each other. The bosses with which the eggs are studded are not mere structural excrescences of the shell, but are pockets containing small masses of a substance which is possibly of service in enabling the eggs to regain lost moisture.

"(3) Eggs on a water surface are usually deposited so close to the margin as to become stranded by capillary action on the sides of pools.

"(4) Incubation seems to invaribly follow laying within 30 to 40 hours, but the hatching of any given batch may be distributed over a lengthy period.

"Cooling to the extent of 5° or 10° F. acts as a stimulus to induce the hatching of eggs that would otherwise have remained dormant for a longer period.

"Bacterial action also appears to be an important factor in hatching and in some instances may be essential.

"(23) Eggs are laid on fallen leaves lying in water holes.

"(5) The longest period of viability observed was 260 days. When kept continually immersed, some eggs did not hatch for periods of from two to five months.

"(6) Eggs brought back from Freetown and those laid in England hatched after exposure to 28° and 30° F. for 24 hours; but none hatched after an exposure of 25 days.

"All the eggs of a batch placed at 108° F. for 24 hours failed to hatch.

"(7) The only active enemy discovered was a species of book-lice (*Psocidæ*). Ants seemed strangely indifferent to eggs of *Stegomyia*.

"*Larvæ*.

"(8) The larval period is conditioned by temperature and food.

"Under the most favourable circumstances the larval life is passed within four days; with a scarcity of food it may be prolonged for upwards of 70 days.

"(9) Shortage of food results in the production of small sized adults.

"Well-covered cleanly cisterns require covers of specially small mesh wire gauze (not less than 18 x 18) as eggs may be washed in from gutters during rain.

"(10) There is an apparent association between the speed of larval growth and the development of bacteria.

"(11) The upper limit of temperature at which larvæ and pupæ may survive lay between 112° F. and 115° F.

"Half the larvæ reared at 80° F. became stiff and immobile at 50° F., irrespective of size.

"At 40° F. all the larvæ became immobile at the bottom of a large tin, and nearly all the pupæ, which remained at the top, also lost all power of movement, but the large majority of both larvæ and pupæ recovered when the temperature was allowed to rise.

"(12) When submerged in a wire gauze tube of 18 x 18 mesh, for 20 hours, 8 per cent. of the larvæ and 27 per cent. of the pupæ survived.

"(13) The larger larvæ of *S. fasciata* apparently consume the smaller ones.

"*Adults*.

"(14) Adults in captivity were observed to pair and feed at any hour of the day or night, late afternoon being perhaps most favoured.

"A single male may serve ten females more or less effectually, and fertilise 750 eggs.

"(15) A single full meal of blood is sufficient for egg production in many cases, possibly for all, though the eggs are sometimes retained for many days before being laid under these circumstances.

"(16) Females in their period of greatest vigour tend to develop and lay their eggs in masses at about three-day intervals, feeding on the first and second days after depositing their eggs, and fasting while the ovaries are full.

"One female laid 837 eggs in twelve batches, exclusive of odd eggs; another laid 712 eggs in fifteen batches during 22 days.

"(17) The kitchen and boys' quarters are the places most often chosen for the deposition of eggs.

"(18) Eggs are not laid by fertilised females regularly fed on human blood except on wet surfaces or on water.

"(19) A female lived for 95 days and was then killed by ants. The longest life of a male was 50 days.

"(20) No evidence was obtained that *S. fasciata* can habitually, or is likely, save under very exceptional circumstances, to tide over the dry season in the adult stage.

"(21) *S. fasciata* probably suffers more from wingless than winged foes once it has gained entrance to a dwelling. This is owing to its retiring habits.

"Ants proved to be deadly foes to caged mosquitoes.

"Two species of spiders in the mosquito house practically lived on *S. fasciata*.

"A small flattened scorpion ate large numbers of adults confined in the same box with it, and a slender wall haunting lizard quickly cleared a large cage of *S. fasciata*.

"(22) The only parasites encountered were a gregarine *Lankasteria culicis* Wenyon and a species of yeast.

General Observations.

"(24) The early tornadoes, which herald the breaking of the dry season, begin as dry squalls with but little rain, and may bring mosquitoes from the outlying districts into Freetown.

"(25) At the onset of the rains breeding is necessarily restricted to a few pools in favourable situations; these should be scheduled and treated at short and regular intervals at the very commencement of the rains.

"(26) Emulsions of soft soap and petroleum in combination are more effective larvicides than when used separately, and with naphthalene added kill all larvæ and pupæ at a strength of 1 in 20,000.

"Petroleum and soft soap emulsion at 1 in 8,000 is not effective in killing larvæ within submerged eggs, but causes many of the less resistant eggs to hatch at once, when the young larvæ are killed.

"(27) Salt water (from Freetown Harbour) speedily kills the larvæ of *S. fasciata*, but does not destroy the pupæ.

"Although it does not destroy the eggs it causes a high percentage of the less resistant ones to hatch at once, and a considerable percentage of the specially resistant.

"The young larvæ after hatching are speedily killed by it. The use of salt water for flushing culverts and gutters, and watering roads might, if practicable, prove very beneficial.

"(28) Adult mosquitoes of normal size were not observed to pass through 16 x 16 wire gauze, but there is little doubt that the dwarf specimens caused by scarcity of food could do so. A mesh of not less than 18 x 18 is essential for safety."

Mr. Bacot sent home some dried leaves of the West African cotton-wood tree, on which were eggs of *Stegomyia fasciata*. These leaves were entrusted for examination to Mr. Malcolm Evan MacGregor, of the Wellcome Bureau of Scientific Research, and a full account of his results is contained in a paper entitled "Notes on the Rearing of *Stegomyia fasciata* in London" (in the "Journal of Tropical Medicine and Hygiene" (No. 17, Vol. XVIII., pp 193-196). The leaves had been a fortnight in transit and had remained in a box at the Colonial Office for three months; nevertheless, when placed on tap water in glass containers, and kept at a temperature of 18° C., crowds of larvæ hatched out between 11.30 a.m. on April 29th, 1915, and 9.30 a.m. on the next day. About 75 per cent. of the eggs had been observed to be dried up, with their shells crinkled and shrivelled, whilst the rest appeared to be normal, yet the number of larvæ produced convinced Mr. MacGregor that the shrivelled eggs, as well as the normal, had been viable. They were kept in water in containers contaminated with straws from horse manure, and the organic matter and bacteria thereon, and were found to flourish best in water at a temperature of from 23° to 26° C.

On emergence the male and female mosquitoes were transferred to a cage, and mating took place usually in mid air.

The female mosquitoes readily fed on a black guinea-pig, and showed a marked preference for an animal of that colour. When a white guinea-pig was substituted the one or two which settled upon it, even when the hair on the back was shaved, were instantly disturbed by the slightest movement of the animal, and flew off to the far end of the cage and remained there, whereas by no amount of movement was a black guinea-pig able to dislodge them.

The males under the conditions obtaining in the laboratory lived between ten days and three weeks, whilst the females lived from a month to six weeks, and some have lived for nearly three months.

For the complete account of these interesting observations, the reader is referred to Mr. MacGregor's paper. We must here be content to record his conclusions:—

> "By the demonstration once more of the remarkable resistance of the eggs of *S. fasciata* to desiccation, attention is called again to the fact of what this may mean, very easily mean, in the distribution of this mosquito, and hence its bearing on the spread of yellow fever.

"It is clearly conceivable that dried leaves with the eggs attached might by wind alone be spread over immense distances, while by export of raw materials in bales of all sorts, dried leaves with eggs adhering could very well be distributed to the ends of the earth. Moreover, the hardiness of *S. fasciata* would permit of its establishing itself in many places where it is not found to-day, and with the sector of yellow fever present the living virus—if such it prove to be—need only be introduced into the infested area for the danger of an epidemic to be made manifest."

MOSQUITOES ON BOARD SHIPS.

At the request of the Commission a careful examination was made of vessels of every class trading to various ports, with a view to determining the presence, and, when present, the degree of prevalence, of the *Stegomyia* mosquito, both in the larvæ and adult stage.

The third volume of the Investigators' Reports contains an account of this investigation as carried out at Freetown, from the 8th April to the 24th May, 1914.

Twelve ships were boarded and examined, but in only three were mosquitoes found.

In the first of these, the s.s. "Patani," which made a voyage from Freetown to Sherbro and back, twenty-four mosquitoes were captured, and identified as follows:

Culex decens	12
Pyretophorus costalis	11
Ochlerotatus (? sp.)	1

It appears probable that they had come on board when the vessel was lying in the Sherbro River, about 400 yards from the mangrove swamps which there line the river.

The second vessel, the "Henrietta Woermann," had come from Assinie, and had touched at eleven ports, the last before Freetown being Sherbro Island, where the mosquitoes probably came on board, as at all the other ports the vessel had not been nearer to the shore than half-a-mile.

Two mosquitoes caught were *Culex duttoni*, both females.

The third vessel was the s.s. "Warri," from Sapeli and Warri. This ship had touched at thirteen ports on the coast, but at all except the two first named she had lain at least a mile and a half from the shore. The ship had been nineteen days on the voyage from Sapeli, and sixteen days from Warri. Identification showed the captured mosquitoes to be:—

Culex duttoni	3
Stegomyia fasciata	1
Culex pipiens	2
Culex (? *pipiens* type)	6
Culex (? sp.)	1

All the mosquitoes were females, except the *Stegomyia;* this was captured in the cabin of the second officer.

Mosquitoes were not found in the holds of any of the vessels examined.

The places on the coast named by the sailors as most infected with mosquitoes were:—

1. Forcados and the various creeks thereabouts.
2. Opobo and its creeks.
3. Benin.
4. Brass.
5. Okrika.
6. Port Harcourt.

The two latter were mentioned by all as the worst. As soon as the vessel gets out to the open sea the mosquitoes almost invariably disappear, but in calm weather, and when keeping near the coast, they may remain on board for many days.

The great variation in the extent to which vessels sailing up these infected creeks are troubled by mosquitoes is interesting to note. For instance, those on board the s.s. "Warri" were greatly tormented by them; whilst the s.s. "Boma," which covered exactly the same ground about ten days later, was hardly troubled at all. Possibly the presence or absence of wind or the direction from which it is blowing, may account for this more or less.

Amongst the twelve ships there were fourteen cases of illness, as follows:—

Malaria	9
Yellow fever	1
Intestinal disorder	1
Pyrexia of uncertain nature, with headache	3
	14

Two cases died, one, according to the ship's surgeon, of Malaria and hyperpyrexia, and the other was the case of Yellow Fever. The latter patient was taken ill and after five and a half hours' illness, died. The vessel, the "Nembe," was then at Burutu.

Assuming that these results, as regards mosquito transference fairly represent what usually happens along the coast at that period of the year, they do not indicate that steamships are then to any considerable extent responsible for conveying mosquitoes from one part of the coast to another; one male *Stegomyia* was not a great catch.

PART IV.

SYNOPSIS.

SECTION I.

ENDEMIC FOCI AND ENDEMIC AREAS OF YELLOW FEVER IN WEST AFRICA.

The Commission favour the view that in that portion of West Africa which extends from Senegal in the north to the French Congo in the south there are always some areas in which the infection is temporarily manifesting itself, and in this sense the West Coast is an endemic area. It is also probable that there are localities or areas in which the infection is more permanent or from which it is never wholly absent. This view is in opposition to that which regards Yellow Fever as a disease of almost universal prevalence in that region.

If this former view is correct, it is obviously of the greatest importance to locate these foci and areas, as until this is done and adequate measures of sanitation are adopted, it is highly improbable that the disease will ever disappear from the country as a whole.

We have already seen how in the past communities have resisted the acknowledgment of infection with Yellow Fever, and it is not likely that their opposition to the inclusion of their locality in a "black list," implying the continued presence therein of that disease, will be any less strenuous now; more particularly as they will be able to point out that the existence of any such foci is a matter of theory and not of fact, and they will possibly urge that, although the disease may have been present at a particular place in which they are interested in the past, it cannot be proved to be there at the present moment.

The Commission have shown by much evidence that, in the past, this disease has again and again appeared in certain places, and that it continues to manifest its presence from time to time in those localities, and also that there is no evidence of its introduction from without as each successive sporadic or epidemic outbreak occurs, and from this evidence they have been led to the conclusion that these areas are responsible for its continued presence in the various Dependencies concerned; holding this opinion they conceive it to be their duty to give effect to it.

Sierra Leone.

Sierra Leone was undoubtedly at one time the most important focus of distribution of Yellow Fever on the West Coast of Africa, but, owing in part to improved sanitary conditions, it has long since ceased to deserve that evil reputation.

In a discussion held in the Section of Tropical Diseases at the annual meeting of the British Medical Association in 1903 (B.M.J., September 20th, 1902), a medical man, well acquainted with the Colony, stated that he had never seen a case of Yellow Fever in Sierra Leone, nor had his predecessor. This statement of fact may be accepted, but history hardly supports what immediately follows, viz., that "if Yellow Fever ever existed on the West Coast of Africa, in all probability it was imported from the West Indies"; or that of a subsequent speaker, who "thought the existence of Blackwater Fever on the West Coast of Africa was greatly responsible for the notion that Yellow Fever prevailed there."

The last epidemic at Freetown was in 1910 (*vide* Second Report, p. 110), since that date no cases have been recorded in Freetown; but in 1914 a patient infected at Boia, 60 miles distant by rail, was removed to Freetown, and recovered after a moderately severe attack (*vide* p. 79).

There is therefore no longer reason to regard Freetown as an endemic focus.

SENEGAMBIA.

The history of Senegambia certainly justifies the conclusion that the following places in that region should be regarded as endemic foci or areas:—

(i.) Dakar.
(ii.) Goree.
(iii.) Rufisque.
(iv.) Bamaku, in Upper Senegal.
(v.) Louaga, and other places on the Dakar-Saint Louis Railway, mentioned on p. 46 of the Second Report of the Commission.
(vi.) Various places on the Thiès-Kayes Railway, mentioned on the same page.
(vii.) Dinguira and Satadougu, in Upper Senegal and the Niger Territories.

The evidence as regards the above places is fully set out in the Second Report of the Commission, pp. 43 to 47.

PORTUGUESE GUINEA.

The Bissagos Archipelago.

The following extracts from the Second Report of the Commission are of importance: "At Bissau Island and Boulama it is stated that cases of Yellow Fever have occurred which did not come under official notice;" also, "It appears that 'epidemics are constantly occurring' at Bissau;" also, "The close attention of the Government of Portuguese Guinea should certainly be given to the sanitary condition of the Colony and the Islands, as they may be a source of danger to other Colonies on the West Coast." It was from Boulama that the disease acquired the name of "Bulam Fever." Bissau Island and Boulama are probably endemic areas and, possibly, very important ones.

The evidence as regards Portuguese Guinea is given on p. 64 of the Second Report of the Commission.

SOUDAN.

The line of the Kayes-Kita railroad is almost certainly an endemic area.

The history of the French Soudan as regards Yellow Fever will be found on pp. 65-67 of the Second Report of the Commission.

Ivory Coast.

Grand Bassam is certainly open to grave suspicion.

The incidence of Yellow Fever at Grand Bassam and other towns on the Ivory Coast is given on pp. 68 to 70 of the Second Report of the Commission.

Gold Coast.

A full account of the various appearances of Yellow Fever at Accra, Quittah, and other towns of the Gold Coast is given on pp. 70-76 of the Second Report of the Commission.

The epidemics of 1910, 1911 and 1912 are analysed on pp. 115, 119 and 124 of that report.

On reference to the account of the occurrence of sporadic cases (*vide* p. 64) given in this Report, it will be seen that the disease reappeared at Accra in 1913, and at various places in 1914. It has been continuously present in the Colony since 1910.

Northern Territories.

In the Northern Territories there is probably an endemic area in the neighbourhood of Bole. The hinterland surrounding the northern end of the Northern Territories may be the source of infection of Bole on the west, and of Tamale on the east.

The evidence as regards Bole, Tamale and Kintampo is given on pp. 72, 79, 85 and 104 of this Report.

Togoland.

The views of the Commission on the past history of Togoland in relation to Yellow Fever are sufficiently clearly stated on p. 51 of this Report.

In Appendix H. to the report* issued by the Colonial Office in 1913, pp. 103-108, a full account is given of Yellow Fever in Togoland up to 1911 by Dr. G. E. H. Le Fanu. The following table

---

* See footnote, p. 132.

and comments, dealing with the occurrence of twenty-seven cases, are taken from the same report:—

"Besides these cases of yellow fever, two suspicious fatal cases in natives occurred at Sansane-Mangu in September, 1910, and one at Sokode in September, 1911, in a European, who died after a very short illness. As these cases have not been confirmed, they are not included in the following table, which sets forth the details of the twenty-seven cases already referred to:—

"YELLOW FEVER IN TOGO.

Year.	Date.	Sex.		Race.		Died.		Recovered.		Place.	Infected in.	Recorded by
		M.	F.	E.	N.	M.	F.	M.	F.			
1905	Jan. 27	1	—	1	—	1	—	—	—	Anecho ...	Anecho ...	Dr. Külz.
	„ 31	1	—	1	—	1	—	—	—	„ ...	„ ...	„
	Feb. 2	—	1	1	—	—	1	—	—	„ ..	„ ...	„
	„ 10	1	—	1	—	1	–	—	—	Lome ...	„ ...	Külz and Krüger
	„ ?	1	—	1	—	—	—	1	—	Anecho ...	„ ...	Dr. Külz.
	Mar. 23	1	—	1	—	1	—	—	—	„ ...	Grandpopo	„
	April 10	—	1	1	—	—	1	—	—	„ ...	Agoué ...	„
	„ 19	—	1	1	—	—	1	—	—	„ ...	„ ...	„
	„ ?	1	—	1	—	—	—	1	—	„ ...	Grandpopo	,
	„ ?	1	—	—	1	1	—	—	—	Lome-Land	Lome-Land	Dr. Sunder.
	„ ?	1	—	—	1	1	—	—	—	„	„ ...	„
1906	April 23	1	—	1	—	1	—	—	—	Lome ...	Badja ...	Dr. Krüger.
	„ 26	1	—	1	—	1	–	—	—	„ ...	„ ...	„
	„ 28	1	—	1	—	1	—	—	—	„ ...	„ ...	„
	May 3	1	—	1	—	1	—	—	—	„ ...	„ ...	„
	„ ?	1	—	—	1	—	—	1	—	„ ...	„ ...	„
	Aug. ...	1	—	—	1	1	—	—	—	„ ...	Tovega ...	
1907	Mar. ...	1	—	1	—	1	—	—	—	Palime ...	Anecho ...	„
	? ..	1	—	—	1	1	—	—	—	Anecho ...	„ ...	Dr. Günther
	? ...	1	—	—	1	—	—	1	—	„ ...	„ ...	
	? ...	1	—	—	1	—	—	1	—	„ ...	„ ...	
	? ...	1	—	—	1	—	—	1	—	„ ...	„ ...	
1910	Jan. ...	1	—	—	1	—	—	1	—	„ ...	Sebe ...	„
	Aug. ...	—	1	—	1	—	1	—	—	Anima ...	Anima ...	Dr. Zubitza
	„ ...	—	1	—	1	—	—	—	1	„ ...	„ ...	„
	„ ...	1	—	—	1	—	—	1	—	„ ...	„ ...	„
1911	June ...	1	—	—	1	1	—	—	—	Misahöhe...	Misahöhe	Dr. Sunder.
		22	5	14	13	14	4	8	1			

"The table shows a striking rate of mortality (66·6 per cent.), especially among the Europeans (85 per cent.); a marked diffusion of cases over the Colony, from the coast-line to beyond the ninth degree of latitude in the north. No direct connection can be traced between the various outbreaks, and the only conclusion possible is the endemicity of the disease in the native population. Külz (1905) was unable to discover cases among the natives, but it is significant that as time went on cases in natives have been reported, two in 1906, four in 1907, four in 1910, and one in 1911.

"That yellow fever occurs among natives, often in a slight and almost unrecognisable form, is the opinion generally held by the medical authorities in Togo. With regard to this, it is interesting to find Krüger (Annual Report, 1905-1906) referring to the 'massed appearance of icterus, with or without fever, which is very common amongst the natives, and frequently suggests infection through contact by the successive occurrence of it in people who share the same house.'

"Sunder, in an article entitled 'Yellow Fever among Negroes' (*Gazette*, 8th January, 1907), concludes: 'It is to be hoped that the assertion that negroes are immune to yellow fever, which has for a long time been in contradiction with the known facts, may be regarded as finally disposed of. The black race is as little immune to yellow fever as it is to malaria.'"

Cases have since occurred in Togoland (*vide* p. 51 of this Report).

Dahomey.

There is good reason for believing that cases of Yellow Fever are of frequent occurrence in this Colony, although the exact localities which should be named as foci or areas are not known.

Nigeria—Southern Provinces.

Lagos must be regarded as open to grave suspicion. It is extremely probable that mild cases amongst the natives of that town occur without their presence being reported to the authorities.

Abeokuta, or the neighbouring native town of Aro in the Egba State, is an endemic focus; the only other hypothesis it is possible to account for the case of Mr. Brooks at Abeokuta is that the disease was imported from Lagos by rail, of which there is no evidence.

There have recently been outbreaks at Onitsha and at the Engenni Concessions Camp near Degema.

The history of Lagos as regards Yellow Fever is given on pp. 80-118 of the Second Report, and in the Report by Dr. T. M. Russell Leonard in Vol. I. of the "Investigators' Reports," pp. 207 to 307, Warri, Forcados and Burutu are dealt with in Dr. E. J. Wyler's Fourth Report, I.R., Vol. I., pp. 42-86, and Appendix I., p. 187, and Burutu in Dr. J. C. M. Bailey's Report, I.R., Vol. I., pp. 88-154.

SECTION II.

QUARANTINE.

Having regard to the general state of war now prevailing (December, 1915), it is probable that a very considerable period will elapse before the Governments possessing Colonies on the West Coast of Africa will be disposed to consider the revision of the present international regulations respecting quarantine for Yellow Fever.

It is, however, the duty of the Commission to deal with this question, as in a despatch from the Secretary of State to the Governor of the Gold Coast the following occurs:—

"I agree with you in thinking that it will be necessary to wait for the result of the investigation which is being carried out by the Yellow Fever (West Africa) Commission before a decision can be arrived at in this matter."

That despatch was in reply to the following:—

"Government House,
"Accra,
"23rd July, 1913.

"Sir,

"I have the honour to inform you that on the 21st instant a telegram was received by the Acting Colonial Secretary from the Acting Colonial Secretary, Lagos, informing this Government that a second case of yellow fever had occurred at that place, that the first case had terminated fatally, and that Lagos had been declared an infected port.

"This telegram was duly passed to the Principal Medical Officer and the Senior Sanitary Officer for their information, and for their advice as to the action to be taken, and I enclose, herewith, copies of a letter from the Senior Sanitary Officer, and of a minute by the Principal Medical Officer, bearing date the 22nd instant, on this subject.

"Personally I share to the full the opinion of the Senior Sanitary Officer as to the futility and inutility of declaring quarantine against a neighbouring West African Colony merely because two non-immune subjects have contracted a disease which is certainly endemic in parts of this Colony, and is almost certainly endemic in other parts of West Africa. Moreover, it may justly be contended that there is actually less danger of yellow fever being imported from an endemic area at a moment when the existence of the disease is attracting attention owing to its occurrence in non-immunes, than there is at any other time. At such seasons, of course, vigorous anti-*Stegomyia* measures are being adopted, and contacts are being isolated, whereas ordinarily such precautions are not being taken to anything resembling the same extent. None the less, I have ordered quarantine to be declared against Lagos, as failure to do so might, not improbably, cause other West African Colonies to declare quarantine against this Colony. At the same time, I venture to bring to your notice the opinion which my advisers in the Medical Department have expressed on this subject.

"These frequent declarations of quarantine cause a great deal of inconvenience to the general public; they discourage and dislocate trade; they quicken the excessive apprehension with which far too many Europeans already regard the known risks of life in West Africa; and they inevitably advertise the less satisfactory features of our health conditions in a way which cannot fail to be detrimental to the material prosperity of a Colony. If the declaration of quarantine on the occurrence of two cases of yellow fever in any part of West Africa be a real protection to the public health, or an efficient barrier raised against the spread of the disease, all these inconveniences and disadvantages can be accepted with some measure of philosophy; but if, on the other hand, the Principal Medical Officer and the Senior Sanitary Officer are right, and no additional security or practical benefit be gained by our present procedure, it would seem to be advisable to reconsider the whole matter, and to endeavour to persuade the Governments of the French and German Colonies in West Africa to agree to some radical modification of the existing practice."

A Sub-Committee of the Advisory Medical and Sanitary Committee for Tropical Africa was appointed in 1910 to consider the assimilation of the Quarantine Law and Practice of the British West African Colonies, to frame a model ordinance, and to draft Regulations and Instructions in connection therewith.

After consideration of the views of the Governments of the four maritime colonies on the West Coast of Africa, the Sub-Committee recommended the following Instructions in connection with the Quarantine Ordinance and the Quarantine Regulations, both of which latter, *i.e.*, the Ordinance and the Regulations, are contained in the First Schedule of their Report—

"INSTRUCTIONS IN CONNECTION WITH QUARANTINE ORDINANCE AND REGULATIONS.

"1. Every Colony shall as soon as possible notify by telegram to the other Colonies the first appearance within such Colony of recognised cases of infectious or contagious disease as defined in the Quarantine Regulations. Such notification shall be accompanied or promptly followed by detailed information on the following points:—

"(1) The locality in which the disease has made its appearance

"(2) The date of its appearance, its source, and the type which it presents.

"(3) The known number of cases and deaths.

"(4) In the case of plague, whether that disease or any unusual mortality has been observed among rats or mice in the locality.

"(5) In the case of yellow fever, the existence and the degree of prevalence of *Stegomyia* in the locality.

"(6) The measures adopted immediately upon the first appearance of the disease.

"2. The notification and the particulars specified in paragraph 1 shall be followed by a weekly telegram notifying the occurrence of all new cases and by information systematically furnished in such fashion as to ensure that the other Colonies be kept acquainted with the progress of the disease. This information shall be sent at least once a week if practicable, and shall be as complete as possible. It shall, in particular, indicate the measures adopted with a view to checking the spread of the disease, and shall specify what steps are being taken.

"(1) in the way of medical and sanitary inspection, isolation and disinfection:

"(2) in the case of plague, to secure destruction of rats; and protective inoculation of persons:

"(3) in the case of yellow fever, to secure destruction of *Stegomyiæ* and their larvæ in the infected place:

"(4) in the case of small-pox, to secure vaccination and re-vaccination:

"(5) to prevent transmission of the disease to other Colonies.

"3. Every Colony shall immediately inform any Colony within which there is an infected place as defined in the Quarantine Regulations as to the measures which it is proposed to take against arrivals from that Colony or place; and shall, in like manner, inform such Colony as to the modification or withdrawal of these measures. Similar information shall immediately be communicated to every British dependency in West Africa."

As regards Yellow Fever, with which disease they are alone concerned, the Commission do not entertain any doubt as to the wisdom of these Instructions, or as to the necessity for the Government of an infected Dependency affording the information, as described under 1, 2 and 3 above, to the Governments of all other Dependencies on the Coast.

This is, however, not the real point at issue. Regulation I. of the Quarantine Regulations, *inter alia*, defines an "Infected Place," viz., as:—

"Any place where any infections or contagious disease exists. Provided that a place shall not be regarded as an infected place because of the existence thereat of imported cases of such disease, or because of the occurrence of a single non-imported case."

The Quarantine Ordinance is as follows:—

"2. Where a place is an infected place within the meaning of Regulation I. of the Schedule to this Ordinance, the Governor may by order declare such place to be an infected place.

"3. (i) (a) The Governor in Council may from time to time make, and, when made, may vary or revoke, regulations for the purpose of preventing the introduction of disease into the Colony or Protectorate, or any part thereof, from an infected place or for the purpose of preventing the transmission of disease from the Colony and Protectorate into any other country or Colony."

The more important questions which the Commission have had to consider are, briefly:—

(1) What measures, in their opinion, should be adopted by the Governor in Council when *two* cases of Yellow Fever are officially recognised in any Colony?

(2) What measures should be adopted by the Governments of other Colonies on receiving such information?

It may be recalled that the First Report of the Commission, issued at a very early period of their work, contains the following (p. 5):—

b- mittee e Medical Sanitary sory mittee for ical a.

"24. In the report of the sub-committee already referred to (Section 5) some of the problems before the Commission are stated; of these the first is:—

"The nature of the disease which during the years 1910-11 and 1912 has been locally diagnosed as Yellow Fever, and which has been the cause of a heavy case mortality.

"Bearing in mind that accuracy of diagnosis is not at present possible, in the opinion of the Commission that disease was extremely probably Yellow Fever.

"25. The second is stated thus:—

"Was it probably the same disease which is recorded in literature under the name of Yellow Fever as having occurred from time to time in the West African Colonies?

"In the opinion of the Commission the answer is 'Yes.'"

The Second Report of the Commission contained (pp. 5-80) a Historical Retrospect of the occurrence of Yellow Fever (1) on the West Coast of Africa as a whole, (2) of "Fever" in the ships of the British Navy on the West African Station, and (3) of Yellow Fever in the Colonies, both British and Foreign, on the West Coast of Africa.

In that Retrospect it is clearly shown that from 1778 to 1910 epidemics of Yellow Fever, affecting both Europeans and natives, have occurred at various periods and in various British and other Colonies on the West Coast of Africa.

The Second Report also contained a review of the "Health Conditions in the West African Colonies during 1862, a year of Exceptional Prevalence of Yellow Fever." *Ibid,* pp. 83—10 (pp. 106-7

"*Commentary on the Epidemic of* 1862.

"It is evident that about the year 1862 Yellow Fever was a widely spread disease in Africa. It by no means follows, however, that because it was present in a great many centres fifty years ago it is to be found in those places to-day; nevertheless, it ceases to be surprising that from time to time it should reappear in one or more of them or in new centres. Like other transmissible diseases, it requires for its continued presence certain conditions, some of which may fail and so lead to its disappearance, and this in a given centre may be either temporary or permanent.

"So far as these records go there is no evidence to show that it was imported into any African settlement from the West Indies or elsewhere in the year 1862, and we have the statement of the Medical Board, whose report (1884) is given on page 34, that whenever it appeared in Sierra Leone (except in 1872) it was 'the undoubted product of Freetown itself.'

"Like some other diseases, it certainly spreads along the lines of human travel, but these records do not show that in 1862 it was carried from one Colony to another. Also, like other insect-borne diseases, it requires for its continued extension the presence of its intermediary host, and so far as our present knowledge goes it is only by the destruction of the carrier that we can hope to wipe out the disease."

The following also occurs in the Second Report (p. 108) as an introduction to an analysis of the epidemics of 1910, 1911 and 1912:—

"A general survey of the position as regards Yellow Fever in West Africa, immediately preceding and at the time of the first outbreak in May, 1910, at Freetown, may be useful as an introduction to an analysis of these epidemics.

"It is unlikely that a knowledge of the past history of the West Coast in relation to this disease, such as now appears in the Retrospect forming part of this Report, was then present to the minds of many of those concerned.

"The memory of the long history of epidemics at Sierra Leone, and elsewhere, had been buried in a happy oblivion, and much of the information on the subject now available has been obtained since that date.

"On this as on other occasions no evidence was obtained, although careful search was made, that the disease had been introduced by an infected ship from the West Indies or some non-African port, and this remains true of all the outbreaks which have occurred since 1910 in the British Colonies on the Coast."

It is obvious from the foregoing that the caution which characterised the replies to the questions quoted in the First Report, which, as already stated, was issued for special reasons shortly after their appointment, is no longer necessary, and that as a result of their investigations the Commission are able to state without any hesitation that Yellow Fever is an endemic disease of West Africa, using that term in the sense of a *maladie habituelle*, and with the limitations clearly stated in this Report.

These preliminary observations appeared to be necessary in order to make clear, without reference to other sections of this Report, the grounds upon which the Commission base their recommendations as to the action to be taken (1) when one or more cases of Yellow Fever, not imported, are recognised officially in any Dependency, and (2) when a notification to that effect is received by the Government of another Dependency.

The Commission do not share the opinion expressed in the despatch quoted above as to "the futility and inutility" of one West African Colony in which endemic foci or endemic areas of Yellow Fever may exist declaring quarantine against another Dependency similarly circumstanced, although they fully appreciate the inconvenience to the public and the injury to commerce which are entailed by frequent declarations of quarantine.

(1) As already stated, they are of opinion that it is of great advantage that all the Dependencies concerned should be kept fully informed as to what is occurring amongst their neighbours in connection with this disease.

(2) There are Dependencies, *e.g.*, Sierra Leone, in which the disease has either ceased to be endemic or has at any rate ceased to show any signs of activity.

(3) By the introduction of fresh cases of the disease from a neighbouring Dependency new foci or areas may be created in a Dependency in which, although such foci are still existing, a determined effort is being made to stamp out the disease.

(4) It is possible that under certain conditions the necessity for declaring quarantine acts as a stimulus to efficient sanitary administration.

(5) They are, however, of opinion that the recognition of the fact that the disease is endemic on the West Coast of Africa creates a new situation which requires that the existing regulations should be modified, as soon as the cessation of the war renders it possible for attention to be given to the subject.

Recommendations.

The Commission recommend the following procedure in connection with the notification of cases of Yellow Fever and the declaration of a place as an infected place and the declaration of Quarantine:—

(1) On the occurrence of a single case or of two or more cases of Yellow Fever, affecting either Europeans or natives, the Government of the infected Dependency shall notify the Governments of the other Dependencies, British and others, in accordance with the present Instructions 1, 2 and 3 set out above.

(2) On the occurrence of two cases of Yellow Fever, non-imported, either in Europeans or natives, the Government of the infected Dependency shall exercise its discretion as to declaring any place to be an infected place, as defined in the Quarantine Regulations, having regard chiefly to—

(i) the distance of the place or places infected from the coast or frontier;

(ii) the interval, both in time and distance, between the first case and the second, as indicating the existence of a single focus of infection or of more than one such focus;

(iii) the efficiency of the measures already taken to prevent the further spread of the disease within the Colony or Protectorate and the transmission of the disease to any other country or colony.

(3) On the occurrence of three cases of Yellow Fever in any Dependency, the Government shall forthwith declare the Dependeney an "infected place" within the meaning of Regulation 1 of the Schedule of the Quarantine Ordinance.

(4) On the receipt of the information described in the Instructions, as to the existence of one case or of two or more non-imported cases of Yellow Fever in any Dependency, the Governments of the other Dependencies shall exercise their discretion as to a declaration of quarantine against the infected Dependency, having regard (1) to the efficiency of the measures already taken to prevent the further spread of the disease, (2) to their knowledge of the sanitary conditions prevailing in the infected Dependency and the reputation of its administration, and (3) to the probability of the disease being transmitted to their own Dependency.

If it is objected that to give a discretionary power as to declaring a place an "infected place" up to three cases, instead of two as at present, is likely to favour the spread of the disease, it may be pointed out that, speaking generally, medical and sanitary administration is becoming increasingly efficient and the recognition of cases correspondingly more accurate; and also that the larger number is a presumptive indication, either of the existence of more than a single focus, or that the outbreak has not been brought under efficient control.

Moreover, many declarations of quarantine would have been obviated by the change recommended, and the experience of the last few years has shown that no harm would have resulted had it been in force during that period. It may be pointed out that the suggested change does not limit the powers as to a declaration of quarantine by the non-infected Dependencies; it merely allows the exercise of their discretion.

There is no doubt that, in the past, cases of Yellow Fever have been concealed in order to evade the necessary declaration of infection, and that at least one of the Governments concerned, whilst declaring quarantine according to the present regulations, has established a land cordon against its neighbours contrary to the regulations dealing with the adoption of that measure.

Possibly any Power which has acted thus in the past will continue to act in the same manner, but this should not, in the opinion of the Commission, prevent the adoption by the British Dependencies of less stringent regulations which, at least as between each other, they may feel certain will be honourably administered.

SECTION III.

SUGGESTIONS FOR FURTHER RESEARCH.

It may be of service to indicate the directions in which, in the opinion of the Commission, further research in connection with Yellow Fever may usefully be undertaken.

Appendix III. of this Report contains the outlines of a scheme for a systematic research on Yellow Fever, for which the Commission are indebted to Dr. A. Connal, Director of the Medical Research Institute, Lagos, and one of their Investigators. The Commission have decided to print it as an illustration of the kind of research which it had been their intention to prosecute had their labours not been interrupted by the War.

Clinical.

(1) Amongst the "General Conclusions" in their Second Report the following occurs: —

> "The mild nature of the attack in certain cases of yellow fever makes the identification of such cases a matter of great difficulty. It is therefore essential that in the future all cases of fever should be carefully observed and classified in order that, so far as possible, such mild cases of yellow fever may not pass unrecognised."

(2) Also the following: —

> "The attention of all workers at this subject should be specially directed to the discovery of a clinical test for yellow fever."

(3) The diagnostic value of the presence of bile-stained casts in the urine in Yellow Fever.

The Commission are still of opinion that all possible methods should continue to be employed in the clinical study of the disease.

Epidemiological.

(4) The nature of epidemics of disease simulating Yellow Fever occurring in the interior of the country and giving rise to considerable mortality.

(5) The existence of new endemic foci and endemic areas of Yellow Fever.

Pathological.

(6) The nature of the jaundice, whether hepatogenous or hæmatogenous.

(7) The value of Da Rocha-Lima's observations on the zonal arrangement of areas of necrosis in the liver.

The value of Palacio's observations.

The Blood.

(8) The diagnostic value of a high hæmoglobin index in the first three days of a case of Yellow Fever.

(9) The differential leucocyte count in Yellow Fever.

(10) The diagnostic value of the changes in the leucocytes described by Dr. J. M. O'Brien (*vide* p. 218).

The Urine.

(11) Chemistry of the urine in Yellow Fever.

Diagnosis from Malaria.

(12) The association of Malaria and Yellow Fever, and the significance of the absence of Malaria parasites and of pigmented leucocytes in cases of fever assumed to be due to Malaria.

(13) The occurrence of albuminuria in Malaria, apart from any urethral affection.

(14) The incidence of the Bilious Remittent Type of Malaria in West Africa. Whether more often a primary or a secondary manifestation of Malaria.

Diagnosis from Uto-Enyin.

(15) The nature of the disease known as Uto-Enyin and by other names.

(16) The occurrence of yellow pigmentation of the nails in Yellow Fever and in Uto-Enyin.

Mosquito Transmission.

(17) Repetition of the experiments of Marchoux and Simond on the hereditary transmission of the virus from one generation of mosquitoes to another.

(18) The changes which the virus may undergo in the mosquito.

(19) Whether other varieties of the genus *Stegomyià* besides *S. fasciata* are capable of transmitting the disease.

The Virus of the Disease.

(20) The nature of the virus, and, generally, the means by which the continuity of the disease is maintained on the West Coast of Africa, either (1) by man, or (2) by the mosquito, or (3) by animals.

SECTION IV.

GENERAL CONCLUSIONS.

In the three Reports already issued by the Commission certain conclusions are stated which, with others contained in this Report, are here summarised for purposes of reference:—

(1) That the following fevers, other than Yellow Fever and Malarial Fever, are met with on the West Coast of Africa, viz.:—Typhoid Fever, Paratyphoid Fever, Pappataci Fever, and (possibly) Undulant Fever and Seven Days' Fever, and possibly also Dengue Fever in a sporadic form, but that there is no evidence of the occurrence of widespread epidemics of any of these fevers in recent times.

(2) That Malarial Fever is the most widely spread of the fevers met with in West Africa.

(3) That Yellow Fever is an endemic disease of the British and other Dependencies on the West Coast of Africa. No sufficient evidence has been obtained that the disease occurs in the Republic of Liberia.

(4) The number of cases diagnosed in the British Dependencies as Yellow Fever has not exceeded sixty in any one year during the last six years, nor one hundred and eighty in all; but the Commission are of opinion that many more cases have occurred.

(5) That probably the continuous presence of the disease is maintained by the existence of endemic foci and areas or otherwise, rather than by its almost universal prevalence amongst the native population.

(6) That the native population is not immune to Yellow Fever, although, as a rule, when attacked, the natives suffer from a milder type of the disease than the Europeans.

(7) That the nature of the virus of Yellow Fever remains unknown.

(8) That there is no evidence that Yellow Fever has been brought to West Africa during recent periods from outside Africa.

(9) That epidemics of a disease have occurred in other parts of Africa presenting some features of a character similar to those met with in Yellow Fever, and that in these epidemics the mortality amongst the natives appears to have been much greater than usually now occurs when natives of the Dependencies on the West Coast are attacked by Yellow Fever.

(10) That a disease of uncertain nature, known to the natives by various names, as for example, Bayloo, Uto Enyin, or Yellow Eyes, prevails in certain Dependencies, usually at a distance from the coast.

(11) That the knowledge of the diseases, other than Malaria, common amongst the natives, both children and adults, inhabiting the "bush" is very defective.

The Commission feel that it is hardly necessary to emphasize the prime importance of a vigorous prosecution of anti-mosquito measures against all mosquito-borne diseases.

SECTION V.

ACKNOWLEDGMENTS OF ASSISTANCE.

The Commission desire in conclusion to acknowledge the great assistance they have received from those gentlemen named on pp. 2, 3 and 4 of this Report, who kindly attended their meetings and placed their knowledge of Yellow Fever, and other matters cognate to the inquiry, at their disposal. Also to the others there named, and particularly the appointed Investigators, all of whom carried out the inquiries entrusted to them with marked ability and zeal.

The thanks of the Commission are also due to Dr. Harald Seidelin for assistance in seeing through the press Volumes I. and II. of the Investigators' Reports.

The Commission have received much assistance from many members of the West African Medical Staff, to whom also they tender their grateful thanks.

The Commission desire to repeat here their appreciation of the valuable services rendered to them at the commencement of their inquiry by Dr. T. F. G. Mayer, West African Medical Staff, the first Medical Secretary, who returned to West Africa at the conclusion of his period of duty as staff officer attached to the Colonial Office.

Dr. H. Lynch Burgess, West African Medical Staff, who succeeded him, took up the work, and continued to the close of the inquiry to perform his duties to the very great satisfaction of the Commission. All the records of the Commission were kept by Dr. Burgess in a manner which greatly facilitated reference to the various papers and reports as they were required from time to time. The Commission desire to bring the services of Dr. Burgess to the notice of the Secretary of State.

To Mr. Alexander Fiddian, their Secretary, the Commission are specially indebted for his unvarying courtesy and for the sound judgment which he has shown at all times during the progress of their work. Mr. Fiddian's advice and assistance have throughout the enquiry proved of the greatest service to the Commission.

JAMES KINGSTON FOWLER.
W. J. SIMPSON.
RONALD ROSS.
W. B. LEISHMAN.
ANDREW BALFOUR.

ALEX. FIDDIAN,
Secretary.

31*st March*, 1916.

APPENDIX I.

ON YELLOW FEVER.

BY L. G. CHACIN ITRIAGO, M.D. (VENEZUELA), M.R.C.S., AND L.R.C.P. (LOND.).

At the suggestion of the Chairman of the Yellow Fever Commission, I have put in writing the observations I have made and the conclusions at which I have arrived from my experience of Yellow Fever in Venezuela.

I regret not to have at hand the numbers of "Gaceta Médica de Caracas" ("The Medical Gazette of Caracas") where I have published two articles on this subject.

Preliminary remarks.—As compared with European towns, the towns of Barcelona, Piritu, Clarines, Anoto and Zaraza are quite small. Their relative position to each other, and to the sea, is given in the annexed diagrammatic map.

Venezuelan country is true country, with plenty of woods and only scattered houses.

By the word *natives* I mean all inhabitants of the country born in it. They are divided into two groups:—

1. The Indian or original inhabitants.
2. The white people, descendants of European—mainly Spanish —races.

Malaria prevails in Barcelona, Zaraza, Clarines, and Onoto, but much more intensely in the last two; which are also smaller than the first two.

In Barcelona and Zaraza Malaria is mainly observed in the outskirts. In Clarines and Onoto Malaria is seen with the same intensity all over the town; perhaps this is due to the fact that both are narrow towns, which means that all the houses are near the open country in two directions.

From 1901 to 1909 I practised in Clarines, with occasional short absences to Zaraza, Onoto, Barcelona, and Piritu. In the course of the year 1907 there was an outbreak at Clarines of what may be called typical Yellow Fever, which at the same time was ravaging the towns of Barcelona, Zaraza, and Onoto. I was struck by the fact that at Clarines the disease was only to be seen in children. and the same fact was observed in Barcelona and Zaraza. The only adults who caught the disease were :—

1. Those coming from some of the neighbouring towns, villages, or country.
2. Those whose residence in the town was less than five years.

In Onoto the disease did not respect any age; both children and adults were equally attacked.

After careful inquiries I found that about 25 years ago an epidemic of *vómito negro* (black-vomiting = Yellow Fever) had ravaged the town of Clarines, and that from time to time there were observed special cases of fever which the practitioners labelled pernicious malaria.

From what I saw during my eight years' experience, as well as from the results of my inquiries, I arrived at the following conclusion :—

In the town of Clarines and at intervals of from five to seven years there are epidemics of the mild form of Yellow Fever, which is called "fièvre bilieuse inflammatoire." These epidemics have been going on unrecognized and labelled Malaria, as this last disease is extensively prevalent, and the practitioners in malarious countries are too much inclined to see Malaria at the bottom of all febrile and even non-febrile complaints. Most of the cases are very mild, but a few assume a serious character and are accompanied by brown or black speckled vomiting, hæmorrhages from the gums, or nose, or elsewhere, and other well-marked signs of Yellow Fever. These last cases are labelled pernicious Malaria. Of course, this does not mean that there are no cases of pernicious Malaria; as a matter of fact, though not so often as most practitioners are inclined to think, pernicious Malaria is to be seen in the town, but the features are quite different.

As the town of Clarines is a small one and the coming in of non-immune persons is very limited, the disease ceases after attacking all susceptible individuals, but it remains latent, I do not know under what conditions, to be aroused afresh when new human material (all born since its last appearance) is available, and certain unknown conditions present themselves.

Every twenty or more years, and under certain conditions, the epidemics assume a very serious character.

Even the most characteristic cases of Yellow Fever, where there is no room for the least doubt, some practitioners label Malaria, partly on the ground that text-books—written when our knowledge of Yellow Fever was in its infancy—state that Yellow Fever is frequent in adults and rare in children!

On no other ground than that stated above, which is based mainly on first-hand knowledge can we explain why, in certain parts, Yellow Fever is only to be seen in children, while in others, both children and adults are equally liable to it.

In my opinion, it is almost certain that the town of Onoto had never previously been visited by Yellow Fever. Probably, in the future, the behaviour of the disease there will be the same as in Clarines.

Country immunity.—I had occasion to see for myself that Yellow Fever is not to be found in the country districts. The only cases I saw in the country were imported from the town, and the disease did not spread. It was only necessary to reside a little away from town to be quite free of the disease.

Racial susceptibility and racial and climatic immunity.—As far as my experience teaches me, special racial susceptibility to, and racial or climatic immunity against Yellow Fever are non-existent. In this respect there are no differences whatever between Europeans and Natives. In those regions where Yellow Fever is endemic the Natives do not acquire the disease, for the simple reason that they have had it before. The inhabitants of those parts of Venezuela (both white and Indians) where Yellow Fever is unknown, are as liable to it as the Europeans. This is an undisputed fact.

If Europeans come into a town at a time when a mild form of Yellow Fever is prevailing, and if they do not take measures to prevent themselves from being bitten by mosquitoes, they will probably develop a mild form of the disease and will become immunized, as happens with Natives.

Clinical diagnosis and treatment of Malaria and Yellow Fever.—With the exception of the mildest form of Yellow Fever which no one can recognize, and assuming that the possibility of the presence of that disease is borne in mind, Yellow Fever is quite easily differentiated from Malaria and quite recognizable clinically. Of course, I am speaking of the rule and not of the exceptions; an experienced eye will make very few, if any, mistakes. As far as my experience tells me, hæmorrhages (as from the stomach, bowels, gums, nose, etc.) and albuminuria, both of which in a lesser or greater degree are the rule in Yellow Fever, are the exceptions in Malaria. The remission of the temperature about the third day and the rising again about the fourth day, the special aspect of the patient, and the initial frontal headache and backache, are very characteristic features.

It is a well-known fact that once Malaria takes hold of an individual it is very difficult for him to get rid of it, and that unless special measures are taken and thorough treatment is carried out, although the febrile attacks may cease, the disease will remain latent and will manifest itself again and again at the least disturbance which diminishes the body resistances. These are the conditions under which the bulk of the people residing in malarious countries live, and they explain quite readily why a fresh febrile manifestation of Malaria—sometimes mild, sometimes serious—may be aroused by a number of different, often trivial, causes, such as a blow, a fall, a fracture, slight gastro-intestinal disturbances, excesses of any kind, and so on. If a trivial cause is powerful enough to arouse the apparently dormant Malaria, it is easy to understand that this may be more quickly effected and to a greater extent by the great bodily disturbance which must be caused by the incubation and invasion of Yellow Fever.

It is evident that if in a serious case of Yellow Fever the probabilities of cure are, say, 67 against 33, these probabilities are diminished by a simultaneous attack of Malaria; in other words, the added factor, Malaria, will render fatal many cases of Yellow Fever which, by themselves, would not be so. Consequently, if by the careful use of quinine the concomitant Malaria is eliminated, the prognosis will be much better.

In the first cases of the epidemics I have referred to, when I had no practical knowledge of the treatment of the disease and was afraid, owing to the statements in some books, to use quinine in Yellow Fever, I abstained from using it, and I saw a very heavy mortality. Later on, and bearing in mind the above considerations, I added to the treatment of Yellow Fever (which in my opinion should be limited to doing no harm and avoiding drugs as much as possible) the use of two daily intramuscular injections of quinine hydrochloride (from 0·25 to 1 gramme per injection, according to age) during the first three days of the disease. The results were most encouraging, both as to the course and the mortality. The disease was not stopped short as it would be the case in a simple attack of Malaria, but the temperature lessened at once and continued not so high as in the previous cases, and the general condition was greatly improved. But, in my opinion, the quinine must never be given by the mouth because in this way it will not, in most cases, be tolerated by the stomach and therefore will not be absorbed; it will increase the gastric disturbance and the tendency to vomiting; and therefore without doing any good will do a great deal of harm.

Consequently, I am of opinion, that in malarious countries the ordinary treatment of Yellow Fever should be supplemented by the careful use of quinine.

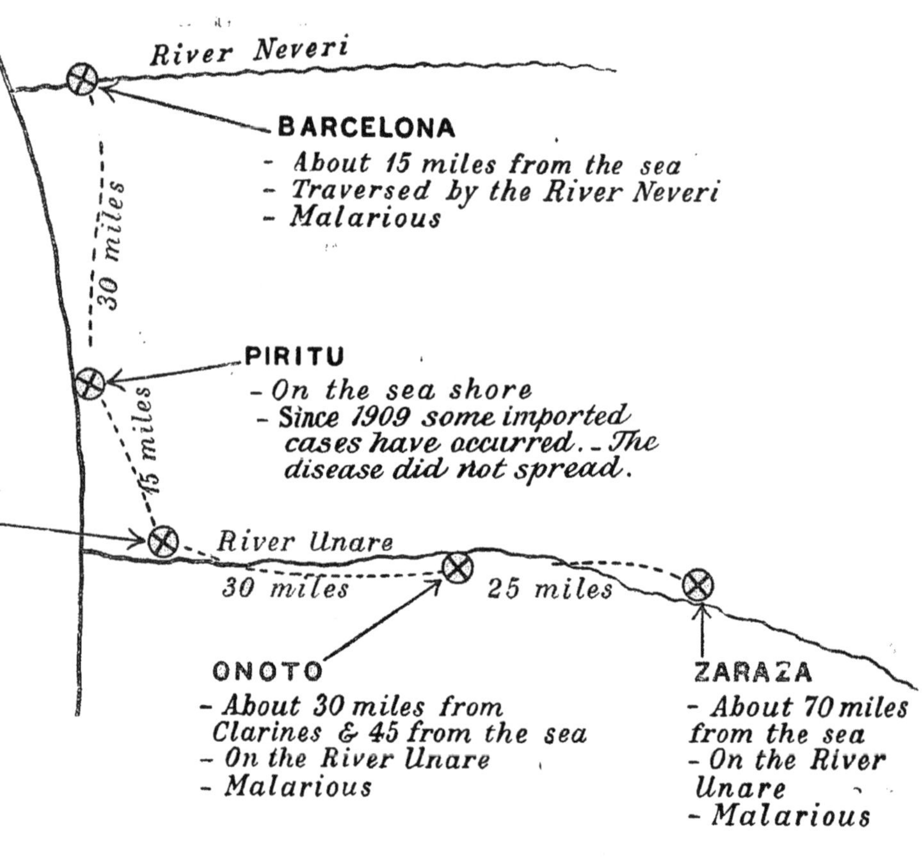
River Neveri
BARCELONA
- About 15 miles from the sea
- Traversed by the River Neveri
- Malarious
30 miles
PIRITU
- On the sea shore
- Since 1909 some imported cases have occurred. - The disease did not spread.
15 miles
River Unare
30 miles
25 miles
ONOTO
- About 30 miles from Clarines & 45 from the sea
- On the River Unare
- Malarious
ZARAZA
- About 70 miles from the sea
- On the River Unare
- Malarious

APPENDIX II.

The Commission print the following paper, which has been abbreviated and put into the form of a continuous narrative, as it is, in the opinion of the majority of the Commission, a unique description of an attack of Yellow Fever by a patient, and brings out in a very striking manner the leading symptoms of that disease. Moreover, the remarks on treatment are of great clinical value.

RECOLLECTIONS OF AN ATTACK OF YELLOW FEVER.

By Alexander Lundie

(Temporary Captain R.A.M.C.; late West African Medical Staff).

On the 6th of September, 1913, Captain Short was relieved at Bole, Northern Territories, Gold Coast, by Mr. Sherriff. A large gathering of chiefs came to welcome back Mr. Sherriff. At night, Captain Short invited me to dinner, but during the course of the dinner my interest suddenly flagged. Everything had lost its taste, and I felt queer. Asking the host's permission, I took my temperature and found it to be 101°. I retired to bed at once, as a matter of precaution.

I slept very well and next day was in exactly the same condition, and kept in bed all day, feeling very drowsy, but quite satisfied with my condition. My host called to say "good-bye," and settle some affairs, and I got up out of bed most unwillingly to get something for him. On returning I felt a stinging at the side of my left knee, and caught a tse-tse fly fastened on the spot. I recognised it easily as *Glossina tachinoides*, and remember being extremely annoyed at it. This was a Sunday morning, and I spent the day and the next two in bed, thinking I had a low malaria. The temperature scarcely varied, and I had no discomfort, and by Wednesday morning I felt justified in getting up early, and going to attend the patients. I had, moreover, many cultures of *trypanosomes* going on, and an interesting *æcidiomycete*, whose life history I was working out. There was also cattle disease, which I looked on as akin to Yellow Fever, and I did not want to miss any chances to dissect a dead animal.

These three days of fever were uneventful, and I was immensely surprised on finishing hospital duties that I had scarcely power to get back to my house. On getting back, however, I took out the microscope and was horrified to find I could not attend to or take any interest in what I was doing. Luckily, the new District Commissioner came over, and distracted my attention, and I put away the microscope. On Thursday and Friday, and the most of Saturday, I made slight progress. No rise of temperature ever took place, but I noticed that I could get a rise to 103° easily by putting the thermometer in my mouth immediately after a meal. This rise was very transitory, and I regarded it as evidence that all was not well, as the greatest rise I could ever get in apparent health on the West Coast in this way was to 101°, and even then I was not sure that there was not some malaria about me, as I was taking quinine very steadily. On Saturday I managed my duties so well that I consented to go out for a long walk with Mr. Sherriff, to the south of Bole. We reached old ruins, which we discussed. Bole had been overrun by Samory, not so very long ago, and it is still full of dead men's bones. We were speaking of these things and our own adventures, when the sun began to set, and we saw it would take us all our time to get home by six p.m. We set out and got on a little way when I said, "I am in for rheumatic fever, and it is a mystery how that should be, as I have not got a chill or wetting at all." I discussed the symptoms and said, "It can't be malaria, at all events." When we got within sight of my house. I gathered my remaining strength and rushed for it, and on arriving shouted for the boy, who helped me to undress, and then I collapsed in the bed and was tucked in carefully by the boy. Mr. Sherriff came over in half an hour and took the temperature and prescribed quinine. The temperature was 102°. The headache was simply appalling, and the pains in the stomach were indescribable. Bilious vomiting commenced, and I decided to have some more quinine and mist. Alba. My skin was horribly dry, and I had grave suspicions that I had not malaria at all, but something incurable, so I took the quinine merely to prove that it was not malaria. I vomited incessantly, but my mind was exquisitely alert, and no sleep came till about 3 a.m., when I was drowsy.

The 14th inst. was dull and uninteresting. At 6 p.m. I had reached 102°, and at 8 p.m. 106°. Mr. Sherriff then took a grave view of the case, and I was startled at 9 p.m. by the arrival of a dozen police with his own bed. Meanwhile, I announced that I had not malaria at all, but in all probability Yellow Fever. I got him to bring me a sealed tube with a solution of quinine in it, and my hypodermic case, and I injected a dose into my flank

I then explained the *rationale* of the proceeding. I said: "This will be my last dose of quinine, if it does not make a very appreciable improvement in my condition in a very short time." I explained that the vomiting might have prevented an effective dose reaching the blood, but the injection would obviate this difficulty, and if unsuccessful, would prove that the disease was not malaria at all. He agreed, and said he would treat me exactly as I desired. That night was spent in the most exquisite agony. The vomiting was so sudden and so urgent that I was thrown violently across the bed in my hurry to turn round and keep the bed clean. Mustard plasters were applied all over me and cold water cloths to the head. Later on in the early morning, I opened my eyes and saw my nurse dozing, and his whole face seemed to be black with mosquitoes. Nevertheless he refused to leave me, when the mere misery of the bites alone would have been sufficient justification for beating a retreat to bed.

Next morning I told Mr. Sherriff finally that I really had Yellow Fever, and would just have to put up with it. I next asked him to wire to Wa, and to Kintampo for help, as he could not go on alone. I then asked him to bring my notes from Sir Patrick Manson's lectures, taken at The London School of Tropical Medicine, and with my own finger pointed out the words: "TREATMENT:—Common sense and nursing. Hot fluid must be supplied as required, but on no account must food be given. The patient won't die of starvation in five days." "Now," I said, "no food for me for five days. And further, no medicine either. You can get a pill box of soda bicarbonate from the dispenser, but don't let him attempt to make Sternberg's mixture, I would rather die a natural death than have perchloride poisoning added to my tortures. The boys can keep the sparklets going all the time as I have bulbs to last a year, and they know how to manage the filter." I then pointed out the following words in my own handwriting, copied from Sir P. Manson's own dictation:—"Mortality varies. 30 per cent. is the average. 50 per cent. to 90 per cent. in an epidemic, or as low as 10 per cent. A drunkard never recovers. A temperate liver usually recovers. If thermometer does not rise over 103°, recovery is invariable. Above 106° F. all die." "Now," I said, "you see I don't drink at all and I have not reached 106° yet." I did not know that the previous night I had done so, or that I was to reach 106·7° in less than 24 hours. This was a very busy day for me, vomiting being apparently incessant, but I had time to notice that everything I saw in broad daylight was brilliant yellow, and was very glad I had diagnosed the case even before getting so broad a hint as that. I was highly alert also, and called my steward boy and scolded him for allowing a hole to wear in the mud floor, and had it filled up at once. That day was really too awful to bear any description at all. About 8 p.m. I was so hopelessly spent that I called Sherriff and gave him instructions how to make normal saline, and asked him to prepare three pints, as I intended to have a rectal injection, slowly, to try to make up for the loss of water from my blood caused by the constant vomiting. I see it has been noted that it took effect in a few minutes. I was never nearer death than then. I had administered it much too fast, and when I got back into bed I seriously wondered if I would ever be able to turn on my back again or would just die on my face. However, I pulled through so fast that I slipped out of bed again that same night and arranged all my correspondence, so that there would be no trouble left for other people who had to look for things.

That night was really the worst I passed. I had been making a new medium from fresh blood serum, and had a good many cultures of *trypanosomes* going on. The Petri dishes I used were claret glasses covered with champagne glasses. I have mentioned that I hoped to recover, as I took no alcohol at all, but I had a full case of wine glasses. These glasses made good media dishes, and I used most of them for that. The tornadoes were in full swing just then, and every night one tore through the house from end to end, carrying away papers and books and smashing things I prized highly. Rain poured through the roof into my eyes every night and added to my troubles. The boys were there on the very first distant moaning of the wind and covered up my bed with a ground sheet, and so saved me from the dripping through the roof, which worried me much more than the fever. The champagne glasses went the way of all the world at that time, and the crash was terrible. They got on my mind, and when I vomited next time, in my delirium, thought that they had stuck in my mouth. Then a calm came. I opened my eyes. It was dawn. My nurse was sitting over me with a bath sponge dripping with cold water. I did not dare to move or sit up. I knew acutely what had happened. I had, in fact, not dared to sit up for some time before, fearing instant death. But I looked around and felt my arms and legs tugging violently. I was horrified. I was in convulsions. I shouted, "Come quickly. Look at my legs. I'm about done. I can't stop these twitchings, and if they don't pass off in half an hour, I will just have to die. Get my keys from below my pillow, and show them to me." He did so, and I showed him the key of the box I wanted opened. He opened it, and got a box of hypodermic tabloids. I said "I am quite clear now, I know I was delirious last night but I am not now. This is my last chance probably, and if I pull through the next half hour I will get better, but it will take some time, and you must not give me any food until I ask it. You will find a tube of morphine hydrochloride tabloids in that box. Each is $\frac{1}{4}$ grain. If you break one into two and give me one half that will be $\frac{1}{8}$ grain. You see I understand perfectly what I am talking about. If the morphine acts, good and well, if not, you can't be blamed." He did as I asked. In 15 minutes I felt easier, and in half an hour felt sure of recovery. Nothing seemed so plain to me all my life as the action of this morphine, and everything that had happened to me in the last few hours.

In spite of my injunctions, I see it in the official report that I was persuaded to take Benger's food twice that very day, but it soon was rejected, and did more harm than good. Another attempt to palm off tea upon me was made late that night, with the same result, but still I felt sure of recovery, and I do not blame my attendant for his endeavour to get me to retain something.

The next two days were dull and uninteresting. Vomiting was so frequent that the resolution not to take food was not defeated. Dr. Mugliston arrived on the second of these days, the 18th September. He had gallantly ridden seventy miles at a stretch through swamps and tornadoes. His transport had been effected by hammock and by our horses. All these unhappy animals have sleeping sickness, and ours were no exception. My horse got washed from under Mugliston's feet into a torrent, and got under a bridge. Mugliston just managed by superhuman efforts to push it out with a stick, and save its life, while he himself stood waist deep on the bridge, to his own great risk.

Next day I took some champagne and Valentine's beef juice, but I did not like either. My urine was exactly like the beef juice, and I shivered to see it, and wondered if I would die in that doleful place, or go home with chronic nephritis.

The morning of the 20th opened bright and cheerily. I was as happy as could be. It was Sunday, a totally different day from all others, even though I did the same work, as a rule. I remember clearly saying, notwithstanding the horror of the previous day, that I would recover without any complications. The 21st passed quietly, and Dr. Watt arrived next day.

Next day I had time to examine myself more carefully, and noted that my fingers had been bleeding beneath the nails and were all black in consequence, and my skin was guinea gold.

I waited on for recovery, having an occasional moment of anxiety when my stomach was rebellious. I drank vast quantities of cold soda water, going right in the face of Sir Patrick Manson's warm drink *régimé*. My "Osler and Macrae" was consulted, and it was found good to give calves' foot jelly and iced champagne. We had none of these dainties. I fed on tinned milk and sparklet water, and managed to use it up. It is absolutely amazing to think what will support human life that is determined not to be put out.

The ten days of my convalescence, from the 20th September to the day I got up, were extremely happy, but I had a few night terrors. A brain so excessively active as mine had been, exercised with superintending my own treatment, could not fail to be tired.

No sooner had I closed my eyes to compose myself for the night's sleep, for the days were unclouded, than visitors arrived. Six other selves, all of them me, sat at my right shoulder on the pillow and worried me with their disputes. They disappeared whenever I opened my eyes.

No doubt this was just at the time when the kidneys were most severely taxed, for it was quite a late symptom. Another night I thought that all the chiefs of the district sat around my bed.

For sheer agony and prolongation of torture Yellow Fever must take first rank. It surpasses rheumatic fever in the exquisiteness of the pains, their variety, and incurability. It is madness to give drugs to relieve them. Any drug able to do it would have to be given in an almost fatal dose. In cerebro-spinal fever stupor sets in, and although the patient goes raving on, he ceases to feel as acutely. Not so in Yellow Fever, he keeps alert till nearly the end. There is a limit to the power to feel pain, and whether it is caused by heated irons, or jagged knives or disease, it ceases to increase beyond that. The sense organs then become exhausted and actually feel less than is going on, but it takes about six days for that to happen. In Yellow Fever, aspirin sodium salicylate and phenacetin never reach the blood or the seat of pain or the brain. They are not absorbed at all. They are not even vomited out, they are shot out with explosive force, and there is danger of rupturing the blood vessels of the brain with the violence of the action. It is cruel to force drugs in through the skin, in the delusion that they may do good. Quinine is useless, and if the blood has been proved free of malaria parasites how on earth can the subsequent giving of quinine be justified? Pilocarpine is worse than useless, as the blood is already too dense, and if the fetish of a moist skin is needful then water must be supplied by rectum. Indeed, it is a wise thing to do. It would flush out the kidneys, and reduce toxæmia, and make up for water lost in vomiting. No water is absorbed by the stomach, but it should be drunk constantly to clean out the blood and acid in the stomach, otherwise there will be dry retching which will soon kill the patient. It is good to put sodium bicarbonate in the water and to have it ærated too, as it neutralises the excessive acidity of the stomach secretion. The headache is intractable by any safe dose of any drug. Cold water cloths help it distinctly. The abdominal pains are peritoneal, and mustard at least distracts one's attention from them. There is much tympanites, and a turpentine and soap enema would do good, and pave the way for a saline infusion. After one good evacuation of the bowels there is no need whatever for another for about nine days, in a bad case, for no food has been taken, and there is no difficulty in starting the bowels with absolute regularity as soon as food is resumed.

When hyperpyrexia sets in cold sponging is excellent. If the pathology of Yellow Fever were constantly borne in mind, the futility of drugging would be realised and many more recoveries than at present would take place. Saline, soda, sponging, and starvation, will increase the recovery rate immensely, and to these I attribute my recovery, for stronger men than I, with a better record of Coast sickness, have gone down with Yellow Fever who might have made a better fight if they had not persecuted their attendant to relieve their agony by some drug or other, and we all know how hard it is to refuse. They should be taught that it is almost certainly fatal, and that any chance they have is in their own hands. They need expect nothing to relieve their pains, or shorten their disease, in the way of drugs, but they will make things very much easier if they will lie still and drink only water, and never worry about food for days on end.

The Sequelæ.—There are no regrets left; no bitterness. The hair falls out, the nails are black and crack and become permanently thin. There are patches of anæsthesia and hyperæsthæsia all over.

In conclusion, I must once again express my gratitude to Mr. Sherriff for his self-denying, ungrudging attendance on me, and for saving my life.

APPENDIX III.

SCHEME FOR A RESEARCH ON YELLOW FEVER.

Attempted Transmission of Yellow Fever to Monkeys and other Animals.

(*A*)—By direct inoculation with blood from a case of Yellow Fever :—

(1) Inoculation of different amounts of blood (amount of blood infective ?).

(2) Inoculation of blood collected by day, and also by night (periodicity ?).

(3) Inoculation of (i) whole blood.
(ii) washed red cells only.
(iii) ,, white ,, ,,
(iv) serum only.
(v) filtered serum only.
} (*Habitat* of virus ?)

(4) Blood collected on different days of illness (duration of infectivity ?).

(*B*)—By indirect inoculation per infected *Stegomyia fasciata* :—

(1) *Stegomyia fasciata* fed on a case of Yellow Fever on different days of illness.

(2) *Stegomyia fasciata* fed (i) by day only.
(ii) by night only.

(3) *Stegomyia fasciata* fed (i) on whole blood.
(ii) on washed red cells only.
(iii) ,, ,, white ,, ,,
(iv) ,, serum only.
(v) ,, filtered serum only.

(4) *Stegomyia fasciata* put to feed on experimental animal at different periods after infecting-feed on patient (length of time mosquito infective ?).

(5) Similar experiments with other common domestic mosquitoes, *e.g.*, *Culiciomyia nebulosa*, *Ochlerotatus irritans*, *O nigricephalus*, *Uranotænia bilineata* (var. *fraseri*), *Culex decens*, *C. duttoni*, *C. insignis*, *Stegomyia sugens*, *S. africana*, and others.

Observation of the Inoculated Animals.

(*A*)—*Symptomatology.*

Attention should be directed to the following :—

Incubation period.
Prodromal signs.
Signs of illness.
Loss of appetite.
Lassitude.
Irritability.
Temperature.
Pulse.
Loss of flesh.
Vomiting (frequent, violent, contents).
Tongue.
Gums.
Jaundice (conjunctivæ, oral mucous membrane).
Stools (frequency, contents).
Hæmorrhages.
Urine (catheter specimen), usual analysis.
Tenderness (epigastrium, liver, spleen, loins).
Enlargement of liver or spleen.
Blood examination (day and night) (cell counts, presence of parasites, degenerations of cells, &c.).
Other abnormal signs.

(*B*)—*Post-mortem Observations.*

Direct examination, and injection into other animals of emulsions of the following organs and tissues :—

Liver. Spleen.
Lung. Heart.
Kidney. Suprarenals.
Thyroid. Salivary glands.
Brain. Cord.
Superficial lymph glands. Bone-marrow.

Animals to be killed and examined on different days of the disease. Fresh smears from and sections of all organs to be examined, and routine post-mortem examination made, noting macroscopical appearances of the various organs and tissues.

Controls.

(*A*) Observations, over a long period, of the normal standards in the various experimental animals in respect of the pulse-rate, temperature, blood, and urine.

(*B*) Observations on the conditions produced by other diseases natural to monkeys and the other experimental animals employed.

(*C*) Inoculation of the experimental animals with blood from normal human beings and from those suffering from diseases other than Yellow Fever, and also with emulsions prepared from organs of various mosquitoes.

(*D*) Examination of fresh and fixed specimens of the organs of mosquitoes of the age and species of those used in the infecting experiments; and of similar material from mosquitoes fed on patients suffering from diseases other than Yellow Fever.

Reservoir Hosts.

Bats are very common in the native towns. Some prefer trees, others the eaves and rafters of houses, but all are more or less domestic as regards their resting-places.

Their habit of sleeping during the day in shady or dark places renders them likely to be the source of the blood-meal of the day-biting mosquitoes.

Blood Cultures.

The blood to be cultivated by various methods and at various temperatures.

Bass' and Ziemann's methods to be employed, with and without removing leucocytes.

Different amounts of glucose and of other sugars to be added to the media.

Addition to the media of bile and of other substances.

Solid media; " N.-N.-N. " medium; ascitic fluid.

Addition to the media of pieces of sterile tissue.

Aërobic and anaërobic cultivations.

Mosquitoes.

Insects used in the transmitting experiments should be bred from ova or from larvæ.

Microscopical examination and injection into experimental animals of emulsions of the following parts:—

Salivary Glands.	Thoracic muscles.
Proventriculus.	Ova.
Stomach.	Larvæ.
Hind-gut.	Pupæ.
Ovaries.	Filtered juices.
Malpighian Tubules.	

Provided that a susceptible animal is found, it ought to be possible, by the means outlined above, to determine:—

(*a*) The *habitat* of the virus, whether in the red cells, the leucocytes or the serum, or whether it is always filterable.

(*b*) When and for how long the blood is infective, and if by day only or by night only.

(*c*) When and for how long the mosquito is infective.

(*d*) Whether any mosquito other than *Stegomyia fasciata* can transmit Yellow Fever.

(*e*) In which part of the mosquito the stage of the virus infective to man occurs.

(*f*) Those organs of the infected animal in which the most virulent form of the virus is found.

(*g*) The practicability of cultivating the virus.

(*h*) The possible existence of a reservoir host.

Sir,

I have the honour to be,

Your obedient servant,

A. CONNAL.

The Secretary,

Yellow Fever Commission (W. Africa),

Colonial Office,

London.

APPENDIX IV.

BIBLIOGRAPHY OF YELLOW FEVER.

The Commission are indebted to Mr. C. J. S. Thompson, Curator of the Wellcome Historical Museum, for the following bibliography of Yellow Fever, made by one of the Assistants in the Museum, from the British Museum Catalogue:—

CARPOT, C. "La fièvre jaune. Epidémie à St. Louis du Senegal." Bordeaux, 1901.

CARROLL, J. "The Transmission of Yellow Fever." Chicago, 1904.

GARNIER, M. A. "La fièvre jaune à la Guyane." Paris, 1908.

HAVELBURG, W. "Die Ursache des Gelben Fiebers." 1905.

SOUCHON, I. "The Mosquito on board of vessels in quarantine ports as a factor in the transmission of Yellow Fever." N.Y., 1902.

SINCLAIR, W. A. "The Aftermath of Slavery. A study of the conditions of the American Negro." Boston, 1905.

CHOPPIN, S. "Importation of Yellow Fever into the United States, 1693-1876." American Public Health. 4: 190.

WOODHALL, A. A. "May it not originate in the United States?" American Public Health. 5: 80.

LICEAGA & RAMIREZ. "Medico-Geographical Views of Yellow Fever." American Public Health. 23: 422.

PHILLIPS, V. B. "Plantation and frontier, 1649-1863." 2 Vols. 1910.

MONTGOMERY, H. E. "Vital American Problems." New York, 1908.

PRICE, J. A. "The Negro. Past and Present and Future." New York. 1907.

ANDERSON, I. "Yellow Fever in the West Indies." London, 1898.

"Prevention of Yellow Fever." Colonial Office Report. London, 1906.

"Report of the Government of British Honduras upon the outbreak of Yellow Fever in 1905." London, 1906.

"Etiology of Yellow Fever." United States of America—Department of War, Surgeon-General's Office, Chicago, 1903.

BONILHA, J. "Contribucad ad estudo de febre amarella." Instituto bacteriologico, Sao Paulo, 1896.

READ, W. & CARROLL. J. "Experimental Yellow Fever." New York. 1903.

JOV, J. " La réglementation de la défense sanitaire contre la fièvre jaune d'après la Convention de Paris, 1903." Paris, 1905.

CARMONA, M. " Leçons sur l'étiologie de la fièvre jaune." Mexico, 1885.

LAWSON, R. " Epidemiological aspects of Yellow Fever." London, 1888.

BERENGEY-FERAUD, L. J. B. " Traité de la fièvre jaune." Paris, 1890.

MARTIN, J. W. " Yellow Fever." Edinburgh, 1891.

LACERDA, J. B. DE. " Omnmicrobio pathogenico da febre amarella." Rio de Janeiro, 1893.

STERNBERG, G. M. " Yellow Fever." 1893.

DAVIDSON, A. " Hygiene of Warm Climates."

JONES, J. " Investigation of the natural history of Yellow Fever."

SANARELLI. " Etiologie e patogenesi della febrė gialla. 1897. Annali d'Igiene Sperimentale." New Series. Vol. VII., part 3.

CUERVO MARQUEZ, L. " La fiebre amarella en el interior de Colombia." Curazao, 1891.

AUGE, J. & PEZET, O. " Epidémiologie de la fièvre jaune—survenue au Dahomey en 1912."

" Bulletin de la Societé de Pathologie Exotique, 1912." Vol. V., page 648.

WHITE, J. H. " The Dissemination and Prevention of Yellow Fever." American Journal of Medical Science. Philadelphia and New York, 1913, c.l. xv. 378.

" The Question of Yellow Fever endemicity in the West Indies." Yellow Fever Bureau. Liverpool, 1913. II. 325.

CARROLL, J. " Remarks on the History and Mode of Transmission of Yellow Fever." Carlisle. Pa. 1903.

Printed by Waterlow & Sons Limited, London Wall, London.

Lightning Source UK Ltd.
Milton Keynes UK
UKHW031555280119
336335UK00005BA/882/P